Elizabeth's Healthy Home Cooking

Includes recipe exchanges for

Crohn's Disease, IBS, Diabetes and Heart Disease

Healthy Cooking!
Elizabeth

Elizabeth Drake Garand

My sincere thanks go to those individuals and groups who contributed their talents to help make this book a reality.

My husband, Andre Garand, proofreader, taste tester, sounding board and supporter;

My children, Haddon Libby, Dan Libby (webmaster), and Julie Benoit who went through the good as well as the bad times when I was ill;

Joan Dubey, typesetting, layout and editing;

Terri Gozzi, proofreading;

Dr. Kurt Isselbacher, Director of the Cancer Center at the Massachusetts General Hospital, Boston, Massachusetts;

Dr. Ronald Green, Chief of Gastrointestinal Disease, Bristol Hospital, Bristol, Connecticut, Assistant Clinical Professor of Medicine at the University of Connecticut Medical Center;

Charlie Gould, a Type 2 diabetic patient at the Joslin Diabetes Clinic in Boston, Massachusetts;

The Joslin Diabetes Clinic in Boston Massachusetts and Connecticut, for all of their expert information and help;

American Heart Association;

Crohn's and IBS Disease Association;

William Robertson, Crohn's patient, and worldwide web site, IBD Sucks, (www.ibdsucks.org), creator for over 11 years;

Len Divenere, Paramedic and Firefighter;

Bob Wollingberg, Pharmacist;

Gary Nathenson, Mentor;

Price Chopper Grocery store;

Sam Vasile, owner and meat expert from South Side Meat Market, Bristol, Connecticut;

Ron Casey, owner of Casey's Fish Market, Bristol, Connecticut;

Gail Bjorkland, chef for Price Chopper Supermarket, Bristol, Connecticut;

Ray Gagnon, photographer, Bristol, Connecticut;

Lynn Allen, photographer for author's photo;

And to all of you that have shared your treasured family recipes with me.

Library of Congress Catalog Number
ISBN 1-4276-0186-0

This book was written, illustrated, and produced by Elizabeth Drake Garand.
Design and layout by Joan Dubey.

DEDICATION

This book is dedicated to my wonderful dad, Bob Drake, a retired newspaper editor,
for always believing in and encouraging me to be the best that I could be.
Dad, thank you for always being there for me.
You stressed the importance of a good education and have been a guiding light in my life.
I am very fortunate to have you as my dad. I love you very much.

This book is also dedicated to an amazing physician, Dr. Kurt Isselbacher.
He diagnosed and treated me as a Crohn's patient;
he educated and motivated me as a person.
He is somehow able to share his enormous expertise as a doctor,
and yet do so in a caring manner.
His patient and gentle care, his real interest in my well-being, and his optimistic
encouragement motivated me to try to help others with this debilitating disease.
I owe him a great debt of gratitude for being an inspiration for the creation of this book.
Dr. Isselbacher, I, and many legions of other patients, sincerely thank you!

"One can indeed manage to lead an effective and productive life with Crohn's disease while we await its cure. Many factors help and certainly diet and appropriate nutrition are among them. The advice provided in this book will serve as a meaningful resource and guide toward that goal."

– Kurt J. Isselbacher, M.D.

Dr. Kurt J. Isselbacher
Director Emeritus, Massachusetts General Hospital Cancer Center and Mallinckrodt Distinguished Professor of Medicine, Harvard Medical School.

Dr. Isselbacher led the Gastrointestinal Unit of Massachusetts General for 31 years. He was Chairman of the Food and Nutrition board of the National Academy of Sciences and a recipient in 1991 of the Bristol Myers Squibb/Mead Johnson Award for Distinguished Achievement in Nutrition Research. He is a member of the National Academy of Sciences, the Institute of Medicine and The American Academy of Arts and Sciences.

Dr. Isselbacher's altruistic qualities make him one of the outstanding doctors of our generation.

"Fear of food is one of the hardest things to deal with when living with Crohn's disease or ulcerative colitis. After a while, it seems like anything and everything you eat causes more pain. Couple this with the body's reduced ability to digest properly what we do eat, and you've got a recipe for mal-nourishment, undernourishment, and the severe weight loss that goes along with them. The recipes in this book are just what the doctor ordered. They've been tried and tested by people with IBD, and approved by gastroenterologists. Not only that—they taste good, too!"

– William L. Robertson

Bill Robertson is a computer support technician at a large university in Boston. He was diagnosed with Crohn's disease in 1969 at age 19. He has run a patient-oriented support forum on the world-wide web for over 11 years, called IBD Sucks (www.ibdsucks.com). Thousands of members help each other get through long dark nights by sharing their experience, strength, and hope with each other, along with a healthy helping of humor as well. Folks from all over the world check in regularly—many on a daily basis—to catch up on each other's lives and welcome the newcomers. Face-to-face gatherings called "SucksFests" occur frequently, often in members' homes. One early member, who was 12 years old when she first joined, just got married and several "Sucksters" traveled to Miami to attend the wedding. This is not at all unusual for this online community. At least 6 marriages have occurred between couples who've met on Sucks, one of which Bill had the honor of solemnizing himself.

"I feel very strongly that the information contained in this book will be of great help to others looking for easy, healthy, nutritious recipes. Elizabeth has also included credibly researched information about nutrition for certain illnesses, lifestyle issues, and food preparation, which can be imple-mented by anyone trying to improve their diet and create a healthier lifestyle."

– Charlie Gould

Charlie Gould is a current patient at the Joslin Diabetes Clinic in Boston, Massachusetts, and a patient advocate medical researcher and writer after personally dealing with multiple cancers for over ten years. Because of his experiences with both diseases, Charlie has a vested interest in cooking for nutrition and health, and is an avid amateur cook.

He has acted as an advisor and content contributor to this book. He also does online counseling for other diabetic and cancer patients, and always emphasizes the important role nutrition and proper food preparation play in day-to-day disease management.

Charlie currently works at Boston University as the Manager of Training in the Administrative Computer Center, and is currently working on several other books. He works and plays well with others, and does not eat his young.

"Having just seen a preview of Elizabeth's book, I am thoroughly impressed with her work. It is clear that Elizabeth's mission to help others to better health is one that has driven her to do an enormous amount of research and hard work. This book will be of great value to those who wish to achieve a healthier and happier life. The great recipes make becoming healthier all the more enjoyable.

I look forward to purchasing multiple copies as soon as it's available. I will recommend this book in my nutrition practice and it will be a very nice gift for friends and family. Great job Elizabeth!"

– Rick Seebauer, B.S.

Rick Seebauer is a graduate from the University of Connecticut, Department of Nutrition and Science. He has spent the past 27 years in private practice as a foods and nutrition expert. Rick also has a business growing and selling organic food.

TABLE OF CONTENTS

TABLE OF CONTENTS (continued)

PREFACE

"Elizabeth's Healthy Home Cooking" was designed and written to be used as an everyday healthier choices cookbook, including recipe exchanges for Crohn's disease, IBS, diabetes, and heart disease. It is meant to inspire, instruct, as well as entertain the reader.

As a child, it was my dream to feed the world. As an adult, I realized that was not possible. A great Chinese philosopher, Lao Tzu, once said "Give a man a fish and you feed him for a day, teach a man to fish and you feed him for a lifetime". As an educator, that was a more realistic goal.

Studies show that only 10% of Americans eat a healthy diet. Today, most of our food comes from supermarkets where we are confronted with row upon row of tempting unhealthy processed foods, precut and wrapped meats, frozen foods, and dairy products. It's important to read the labels so we know what we are feeding our families. Unfortunately busy homemakers are working and wearing many hats and sometimes just don't have, or take, the time to read them. Over the past 5 years, I have attempted to do it for you.

In this land of plenty, cost limits many of us. There is no problem in getting enough food to fill the stomachs and please the palates of our families. However, in keeping our purchases within the limits of our food budgets, are we feeding our families properly? Many of us are not. Even those of us who have studied foods and their preparations have had to learn in our own kitchens practical ways on how to convert relatively small grocery budgets into dishes that are both nutritious and pleasant for our families.

With knowledge of what to buy, when to buy it, and how to put the ingredients together, without missing out on quality family time, you can have healthier diets. In this land of plenty, we have to make healthier food choices and practice portion control.

Within the covers of this book, I have compiled information gathered during my 6 years of college and 28 years of teaching home economics (family and consumer science). Through practical application in the classroom, interviewing experts in the food industry, reading hundreds of books, and from talking to you, the busy homemaker.

Note that all recipes in this book include modifications to also meet the individual needs of people with Crohn's, IBS, diabetes and heart disease.

When calculating the recipe conversions for Crohn's, IBS, diabetes, and heart disease, I used the following products and their counts reported by their manufacturers: Splenda, I Can't Believe It's Not Butter spray, Light Promise margarine, Light Smart Balance, Carbfit soymilk, and King Arthur flour products, to name a few.

I would like to thank the following sources that provided the nutritional counts:

http://www.nalusdagov/fnic/foodcomp, The "NutriBase Nutrition Facts Reference, Second Edition."

Adjust your counts based on what products you use. The counts are estimates.

TIPS ON HOW TO BE A WISE GROCERY SHOPPER

1. Plan a week's menu using the newspaper, store circulars, and internet coupons as your guide. Some of the websites are coolsavings.com, valuepak.com, grocerystores.com and couponcart.com.

2. Make a shopping list and avoid unnecessary trips to the convenience store.

3. Group items as they are found in your favorite grocery store.

4. Watch for triple coupons. The Sunday paper usually carries the most coupons. Many stores will honor competitors' coupons.

5. Shop for food and non-food items separately. Buy non-food items only once a month at discount stores. Buy them in bulk to save money.

6. Take time to do comparative shopping, and read the labels.

7. Never shop when tired or hungry. Eat before shopping to avoid being a compulsive shopper. Shop alone; children and friends will distract you. If you do take your children, feed them first, or bring a healthy snack. Wash their hands with a hand sanitizer before they eat. I carry a small bottle of Purell in my pocketbook.

8. The ingredients on the label are listed by weight in descending order. If corned beef and potatoes are listed as potato, beef, etc… it means there are more potatoes than beef in the can.

9. Watch the scales and cash register to make sure no mistakes are made.

10. The most expensive items are usually displayed at eye level.

11. Don't buy foods on sale if they are unlikely to be used.

12. Go directly home after shopping to keep food as fresh as possible. Store perishables in a cooler in your car.

13. Leave store coupons in a folder in the car so you won't forget them. Store coupons according to expiration dates.

14. When buying baking powder, I make sure the label says "aluminum-free" (see under definitions).

15. If shopping at a farmer's market, plan to go later in the day. Farmers prefer not to take produce home and will sell them for less.

16. Always check the expiration dates on all perishable food items.

17. Local fruit will always be cheaper when in season. Freeze it for the winter months.

18. Make sure that breads and cereals say whole grain, not just wheat. Whole grain has more fiber than whole wheat.

19. Buy fruits and vegetables from the produce discount shelf. Check for bruises. Discount bananas make great banana bread.

20. I avoid ready prepared food mixes containing palm oil which is high in saturated fats. While less expensive for the manufacturers to use, it is less healthy than vegetable oils and sprays.

21. Read the labels, know what you are buying. Sugar comes by many names; dextrose, fructose, glucose, lactose, corn syrup, honey, maple syrup, and molasses. Before putting molasses or honey in a measuring cup, coat inside of cup with cooking spray and sticky substances will not stick.

22. Buy monounsaturated fats such as canola, extra virgin olive oil, vegetable oils and sprays. These are healthier than saturated fats, such as palm and lard. Fats that are solid at room temperature will increase your risk of heart disease and cancer.

23. Buy trans fat-free margarine.

24. Buy meat and other perishable items early in the morning to take advantage of advertised specials. There are fewer people in the store at that time too.

25. Meat in packages not sold the day before will be sold the next morning. They are still good and may be frozen.

26. Buy 93 to 98% ground beef and add about 1 to 2 tablespoons canola oil to insure moisture. Canola oil is much healthier than animal fat.

27. When buying eggs, make sure they are in the refrigerator case and that the small point is facing down.

28. Keep an ice chest or cooler in the car trunk to safely transport perishable items.

29. Buy flour that is unbleached and never bromated. I use King Arthur organic whole wheat or all-purpose, unbleached, organic flour.

WHAT IS CROHN'S DISEASE AND IRRITABLE BOWEL SYNDROME (IBS)?

Shortly after college, I was hired as a high school home economics teacher. I loved the challenge and was working very hard. About six months into the school year, I woke up one morning with terrible pains in the lower right hand side of my abdomen, had a high fever and was living in the bathroom. It had to be the flu. Unfortunately, the flu didn't go away. From that day on, my life was changed forever. I went to my physician and he said it could be Crohn's disease. I had never heard of the disease and wanted a second opinion.

Dr. Kurt J. Isselbacher, a renowned leader in gastrointestinal disorders from Massachusetts General Hospital in Massachusetts, confirmed that I did indeed have Crohn's disease. Dr. Isselbacher explained that the disease was a serious inflammatory condition that involved the small intestine and part of the large intestine. Crohn's disease may involve the entire gastrointestinal track. Mine was located in the ileum.

Where could I have contracted this disease? Unfortunately, the cause and cure are unknown. There are many theories though. It is believed that Crohn's disease and IBS run in families and that one's environment could play a major role in the disease. It has been documented that there are more incidents of Crohn's disease in well-developed areas of the world, such as North America and Northern Europe.

There are fewer cases in southern climates and underdeveloped areas.

People between the ages of 15 to 40 and 50 to 80 are more likely to develop the disease.

Men, women, and children are at risk for developing Crohn's, IBS, and colitis.

Smoking seems to have an adverse affect on Crohn's disease. Having never personally smoked, I did experience secondhand smoke from my relatives.

In regard to diets, there seems to be certain foods that trigger the disease. It may vary from person to person. The following foods journal will help you to decide what foods you should eat. They include: dairy products, red meats, dark meat from chicken and turkey, egg yolks, fried foods, fats, coffee and caffeine, and other products. What bothers one Crohn's patient may not bother another. It has also been noted that Crohn's patients seem to have diets high in refined sugar. There are other studies that say Crohn's patients increase their sugar intake over time. Either way, refined sugar isn't good for anyone. Since I have eliminated refined sugar from my diet, I feel great...have lost a few pounds too!

My fat intake has been lowered by only eating baked, broiled, or steamed foods.

Dr. Isselbacher stressed the importance of plenty of rest and I have found that to be so true.

While teaching, I was so afraid of being sick and having to leave my classroom that I hardly ever ate and never drank enough water.

I ended up with many kidney stones. If you have ever had one, you know how painful they are.

My stones contained oxalates. Some of the foods that are believed to be high in oxalates are rhubarb, spinach, strawberries, chocolate, wheat bran, nuts, beets, squash, and tea.

When I retired from teaching in 2000, I had less stress, and began to eat and drink properly.

IBS is one of the most common intestinal disorders that cause abdominal pain, cramping, bloating and diarrhea or constipation. IBS is a long-term, manageable condition. People that have IBS may develop pain in response to one or more factors including: Eating, Stress, and Genetics. Women are twice as likely as men to develop IBS. The symptoms are believed to be a faulty communication between the brain and the intestinal tract.

The treatment is adapted to fit individual needs and focuses on changes in lifestyle and diet...Like Crohn's and Colitis, (Inflammatory Bowel Disease) there is no cure for IBS.

People with Crohn's disease, colitis and IBS have a tendency to have excessive gas. To avoid gas, eat slowly, eat small meals, chew food thoroughly, don't drink from a straw, avoid drinking and talking while eating, and don't chew gum.

If on any steroids, such as prednisone, taking alternagel, prior to the medication, will protect the stomach from developing an ulcer. It can be purchased at your local pharmacy. Check with your physician before taking any medication or supplement.

The following is a list of foods that seem to trigger Crohn's disease, Colitis and IBS. With the use of this foods journal, you can choose your own list of foods to avoid and better foods choices. Every patient will have different trigger foods. Then create your own list of foods to keep your disease under control.

FOODS JOURNAL – CROHN'S DISEASE AND IBS

FOODS TO AVOID:	BETTER FOOD CHOICES:
whole bran; granola cereals	Rice Krispies; Cream of Rice; well-cooked oatmeal; ground buckwheat (healing properties)
whole bran breads	oatmeal bread; pita; sourdough; Italian (no dairy); small bagels; English muffins
white bread; pastries; doughnuts; biscuits	small bagels; English muffins
processed foods	organic foods
celery	celery powder
string beans, corn, cabbage	French-style beans, cooked carrots, mushrooms
unpeeled vegetables	cooked and peeled vegetables, sweet potatoes, artichokes, pureed tomatoes
garlic; onion	garlic and onion powder, cooked garlic and onions
gassy vegetables	baby food vegetables

FOODS TO AVOID:	BETTER FOOD CHOICES:
rough skinned fruit	cooked and peeled fruit; pineapple puree
blueberries	cooked blueberries; bananas; applesauce; cooked pureed cherries (anti-inflammatory)
prune juice	low-acid OJ; cranberry juice, pineapple juice (after a meal)
palm oil; hydrogenated fats	canola; vegetable oils; olive oils; cooking spray
butter; hydrogenated shortening	extra virgin olive oil; trans fat-free margarine
dairy products	soy milk; dairy substitutes; rice milk
cheese	soy cheese; active culture yogurt
fried food	baked; broiled; boiled
red meat and fat	93% lean red meat
dark meat turkey and chicken	white meat poultry; free-range chicken, beef, lamb (no hormones or antibiotics)
poultry skin	avoid poultry skin
egg yolk (high fat content)	egg white and substitute
fried fish - not farm raised	baked or broiled salmon from Alaska; sole; haddock; tuna in water; lake trout; scallops; crabmeat
coffee	herbal tea and water
popcorn	pretzels, baked chips
nuts	ground walnuts
hot spices	ginger; mint; cinnamon (aids in digestion)
carbonated and caffeinated beverages	water
Baker's chocolate	cocoa powder
cakes	angel food cake
Aspartame (NutraSweet), Saccharine, cyclamate, sorbitol, refined sugar, BHA, BHT, MSG, nitrates, additives, sulfer dioxide	natural sweetener - fructose; stevia; pure maple syrup; natural, wholesome, organic food

DAILY FOODS JOURNAL – CROHN'S DISEASE & IBS

Date: _____

Foods	Sugar	Fat	Carbs	Calories	Sodium	Chol	Reactions
Breakfast							
Lunch							
Dinner							
Snacks							
Daily Totals:							

WHAT IS DIABETES?

Charlie Gould, a contributor to this work, and a Type 2 diabetic patient at the Joslin Diabetes Clinic in Boston, Massachusetts, wrote the following regarding the importance of diet to control the disease. Charlie has been researching the relationship of diet to serious illness for the past ten years. He is a patient expert.

One of the common diseases that afflicts many in the United States and around the world is Diabetes Mellitus. According to information from the renowned Joslin Diabetes Clinic in Boston, Massachusetts, diabetes is the sixth leading cause of death in the US, accounting for approximately 213,000 deaths per year.

Complications from diabetes include severely increased risks, and are a leading cause of heart attacks, strokes, blindness, kidney failure, and lower limb amputations. Obviously, this is a very serious disease. It occurs when the body either fails to produce insulin (Type 1), does not produce enough of it, or the insulin that is produced is not utilized by the body properly (insulin resistance, or impaired glucose tolerance, Type 2), in order to convert food into energy.

This connection with food is vitally important, as you can influence the course of the disease and help to minimize serious complications with dietary changes on a daily, and long-term basis. Some people with diabetes can control their disease through diet and exercise alone, while others may need some sort of pharmaceutical help as well, from the various classes of diabetes medications in pill form, to actual insulin injections.

Since food has such a large bearing on blood sugar levels, Elizabeth researched the ingredients in every recipe in this book, and has included the changes necessary to adjust, where possible, each recipe for those who may be battling this insidious disease.

According to the Joslin Diabetes Center, it's essential for diabetics to do the following:
1. Practice portion control.
2. Eat well-balanced meals.
3. Make wise food choices.
4. Try to eat meals on time.
5. Have diets low in sugar, fats, and sodium.
6. Take time to read the labels.
7. Strive to obtain and maintain a healthy weight.
8. Seek ways to minimize stress.
9. Drink 6 to 8 glasses of water a day.
10. Exercise daily to help with losing weight and staying fit.
11. At least half of your food intake should come from vegetables, fruits, and whole grain products.

Some of the signs of diabetes are:

1. Excessive thirst
2. Frequent urination
3. Weight loss
4. Blurred vision
5. Increased hunger
6. Frequent skin, bladder, and gum infections
7. Irritability
8. Numbness of hands and feet
9. Slow to heal wounds
10. Extreme fatigue

ATTENTION DIABETICS!

All purpose, unbleached, organic flour may be used for diabetics when baking. If choosing to use the recipe exchanges of soy or rice flour, mix in the following combinations: 2 cups rice flour, 2/3 cup potato flour, 1/3 cup tapioca flour. Mix well and keep in an airtight container until needed. Use mixture cup for cup.

Obviously, any diet recommendations, prescription drugs, and other treatments recommended by your health care team come first, and should not be forgone in favor of these recipes alone. But being able to prepare low-cost, nutritious, and diabetes-friendly meals can only help you if you are dealing with this disease, while providing a wide variety of delicious foods!

The following is a list of better food choices for diabetics. I have also provided a foods diary to keep track of what you eat.

FOODS JOURNAL – DIABETES

FOODS TO AVOID:	BETTER FOOD CHOICES:
white bread; enriched flour	100% whole grain bread; pita; spelt whole grain flour
white rice	whole grain brown rice; long grain rice
sugar cereals	whole grain cereals; rolled oats; buckwheat; barley; millet
muffins; doughnuts	homemade healthy muffins
croissant	small bagel; English muffin
seasoned bread crumbs	unseasoned bread crumbs
salted saltine	graham crackers
frozen vegetables with sauces	fresh vegetables; cruciferous vegetables
corn; peas	cooked tomatoes; chili peppers; bell peppers
canned vegetables w/added sodium	low or no sodium canned vegetables
sodium	spices
spices containing salt	ginger; cinnamon; spices containing powder
roasted nuts; seeds; dry roasted peanuts	almonds; pine nuts; sunflower and pumpkin seeds; walnuts

FOODS JOURNAL – DIABETES (continued)

FOODS TO AVOID:	BETTER FOOD CHOICES:
garlic salt; onion salt	garlic powder; onion powder
heavy syrup canned fruits	light syrup or no-sugar-added canned fruit; blueberries; strawberries; watermelon; fresh fruit (especially grapefruits)
hydrogenated shortening	cooking sprays; flax seed oil
butter	trans fat-free margarine
palm oil	canola; extra virgin olive oil; safflower
whole milk	skim milk
processed cheese	fat-free, part-skim cheeses
fried food	baked; broiled; poached foods; tuna fish; scallops; shellfish
egg yolks	egg whites; egg substitutes
fried fish	baked or broiled salmon; filet of sole; haddock; Alaskan cold water fish; lake trout
red meat (beef, pork, lamb, veal)	only 4 oz, three x per week, lean meat, 93% fat-free, free-range, hormone and antibiotic-free (add 1 to 2 tablespoons canola oil to 1 lb beef)
cold cuts; sausage; processed foods	organic, unprocessed foods
hot dogs	white turkey and chicken meat
dark turkey and chicken	remove skin
carbonated beverages	water; green tea
light chocolate	cocoa powder; dark chocolate
potato chips	air-popped corn; baked chips
cakes	angel food cake
Cheez-it	reduced-fat Cheez-it; rice cakes
sauces; gravies	season with spices
ice cream	low-fat yogurt; sorbet
refined sugar; aspartame	Splenda; fructose; stevia
BHA; BHT; MSG; nitrates; additives; sulfer dioxide	natural, wholesome, organic foods

DAILY FOODS JOURNAL – DIABETES

Date: _____

Foods	Sugar	Fat	Carbs	Calories	Sodium	Chol	Reactions
Breakfast							
Lunch							
Dinner							
Snacks							
Daily Totals:							

WHAT IS HEART DISEASE?

Heart disease is a disorder that affects the heart's ability to function properly. It is one of the leading causes of death in men and women.

A common cause of heart disease is narrowing of the coronary arteries that supply blood to the heart. This blockage happens over a period of time. A good healthy lifestyle will help reduce your risk of heart disease and stroke.

The following is a list from the American Heart Association (AHA) of risk factors we should all be aware of, and that we CAN control.

1. Avoid smoking.
2. Keep your blood pressure in check.
3. Have your HDL checked. It's the good cholesterol that protects us from heart disease.
4. Also have your LDL checked. LDL is the bad cholesterol. It's a soft, waxy substance that builds up in the arteries.
5. Obesity.
6. Sedentary lifestyle…exercise 3 times a week.
7. Make wise food choices. Avoid fast food and buffets.
8. Avoid stress.

We have NO control over family history and age.

How to lose weight the healthy way…

Keeping your weight down is essential for a healthy heart. There are no fad diets that work. The fact is, you have to burn more calories than you consume. Rather than eating 3 large meals a day, eat 5 small meals every 3 hours, this will speed up your metabolism. A meal could be one small apple. Make wise food choices, and like diabetics, practice portion control. Eat before you shop, and avoid impulsive buying. Most of the grocery stores today provide us with sample displays of food to taste. You can consume a whole meal before you leave the store. Truthfully, you have to want to lose weight. Change your environment. Get rid of all the junk food in your cabinets, and have healthier snacks, such as, cut up vegetables and fruits. Also, don't eat in front of the TV. Always eat at the same table and use a smaller plate. Don't eat seconds. Drink a couple of glasses of water an hour or 2 before your meals, especially if you feel hungry. The cravings will pass with water.

When shopping, always park a distance from your destination and walk.

During lunch hour, walk.

Avoid eating late at night. Skip buffets and fast food restaurants.

Most restaurants give big portions of food, share with your spouse or friend. Order one meal with 2 plates.

Anna Paternostro, an independent 95 year old, lives alone and leads a very active life. I asked her, "What is your secret to longevity and healthy living?"

The following recipe is based on Anna's answers to me.

RECIPE FOR A HEALTHY LIFESTYLE

Ingredients:

Temp: 98.6°
Time: Lifetime
Yields: Healthy Lifestyle

Exercise for 30 minutes, 3 times a week (walking is good). Physical activities prevent obesity, heart disease, and bone loss.

Adequate sleep (everyone is different, 6–8 hours).

100% healthy eating habits.

Don't skip meals, yet don't overeat.

Replace fats in some recipes with applesauce or other purees.

Limit intake of red meats and eat only the portion size of a deck of cards.

Eat lean fish, haddock, halibut, sole, striped bass.

Take half a Bayer aspirin (check with your physician).

Yearly health exams.

Abundant servings of fruits and vegetables (5–9 servings per day).

Diets rich in antioxidants and beta-carotene to fight diseases.

Buy local fruits and vegetables in season.

Avoid fried foods. Eat baked, broiled, and boiled.

Avoid alcohol.

NO Smoking.

Avoid stress, walking helps.

Drink 6–8 glasses of water each day. (A report from John Hopkins says not to freeze plastic bottled water as it will release a poison called Dioxin.)

Eat whole grain breads, cereals, and pasta.

Avoid white bread, rice, and flour (it will age you).

Eat smaller meals, easier on your digestion. Five to six small meals a day.

Diets low in saturated fats, salt, and sugar (recommended amounts – 0).

Use extra virgin olive oil or canola oil and cooking sprays when cooking.

Use fat-free mayonnaise (made with canola oil).

Avoid sugarcoated cereals, doughnuts, chips, and sweets. Have cut up fruits and vegetables instead. Sugar also ages your skin and causes wrinkles.

Flavor foods with herbs, not salts. Herbs should contain powder, not salt.

Buy margarine that is trans fat-free and reduced calorie.

continued on next page

Recommended intake on a 2,000 calorie diet should contain less than 65 gm of fat, less than 20 gm of saturated fats, less than 300 mg cholesterol, 300 gm carbohydrates total, and less than 2499 mg of sodium. One teaspoon salt is equal to 2,000 mg.

Use lemon juice on salads.

Reduce whole milk with nonfat, or buy reduced-fat milk and skim milk.

Read the labels—know what you are eating. Foods that are low-fat may have extra sugar added.

Remove skin from poultry. Dark meat contains more fat.

Chill meat and poultry broth and stocks, spoon off fat.

Buy cold water fish such as salmon and tuna. Eat fish 3 times a week. Buy tuna fish packed in water.

Use low-sugar jams and marmalade instead of butter on toast.

Avoid overly processed foods.

Eat lots of "cruciferous" vegetables (described later in the book). They are broccoli, cauliflower, Brussels sprouts and cabbage. These are believed to prevent certain types of cancer. Eat fruits and vegetables full of antioxidants and beta-carotene. They prevent damage done by free radicals.

Have diets rich in tomatoes, garlic, citrus fruits, soybeans, berries (especially blueberries, strawberries and raspberries), cruciferous vegetables, whole grain foods and flax. Stop to smell the roses and appreciate what you have.

Directions:

1. Stir the above ingredients with common sense.
2. Sprinkle abundantly with a sense of humor.
3. Stir in quality family time with tons of love and patience.
4. Bake in the sunshine (wearing SPF 15 suntan lotions).
5. Serve daily with generous helpings.

The following is a list of better food choices for heart disease prevention. I have also included a food diary to keep track of what you eat. Check with your physician before starting any diet.

FOODS JOURNAL – HEART DISEASE

FOODS TO AVOID:	BETTER FOOD CHOICES:
white bread; rice; enriched flour	brown whole-grain bread; all-purpose, unbleached, organic flour
sugarcoated cereals	whole grain cereals; whole grain organic flour; buckwheat; barley; millet; spelt flour
muffins; doughnuts; croissants	small bagels; English muffins
seasoned bread crumbs	plain bread crumbs (make your own)
Saltine crackers	graham crackers
frozen vegetables with sauce	fresh vegetables; frozen plain
canned veggies with sodium	low or no sodium added veggies
canned soups with sodium	canned soups without sodium
processed foods	organic, nonprocessed foods
spices containing salt (garlic salt)	spices containing powder (garlic powder)
canned fruits in heavy syrup	canned fruits in light syrup or no sugar; fresh fruits; blueberries; watermelon; apples; cherries; bananas
shortening; hydrogenated fats	cooking sprays; vegetable oils
butter	trans fat-free margarine; heart safe margarine (Promise)
palm oil	canola; extra virgin olive oil; vegetable oils
whole milk	skim; 1% low-fat
processed cheese	fat-free, part-skim cheese
fried foods	baked; broiled or poached
egg yolks	egg whites; egg substitute
fried fish	baked; broiled; poached salmon; sole; haddock; wild cold water fish

FOODS JOURNAL – HEART DISEASE (continued)

FOODS TO AVOID:	BETTER FOOD CHOICES:
red meat (beef, pork, lamb, veal)	lean ground beef, 93% fat-free, range-fed, no hormones or antibiotics (add 1 to 2 tablespoons canola oil per pound for moisture)
cold cuts; sausage	home baked turkey or chicken
hot dogs	turkey dogs
dark meat turkey and chicken	white meat turkey and chicken
poultry skin	remove turkey and chicken skin
carbonated beverages	water; green and herbal teas
Baker's chocolate	cocoa powder; dark chocolate
potato chips	air-popped corn; baked chips
cakes	angel food cake with fresh fruit
sauces and gravies	season with spices
ice cream	low-fat yogurt and sorbet
salt	no salt; use sodium-free spices
refined sugar; aspartame	Splenda; fructose; stevia (from sweeting herb)
roasted nuts and seeds; dry roasted peanuts	almonds; pine nuts; sunflower and pumpkin seeds
BHA, BHT; MSG; nitrates; sulfer dioxide; additives	additive-free, wholesome foods

DAILY FOODS JOURNAL – HEART DISEASE

Date: _____

Foods	Sugar	Fat	Carbs	Calories	Sodium	Chol	Reactions
Breakfast							
Lunch							
Dinner							
Snacks							
Daily Totals:							

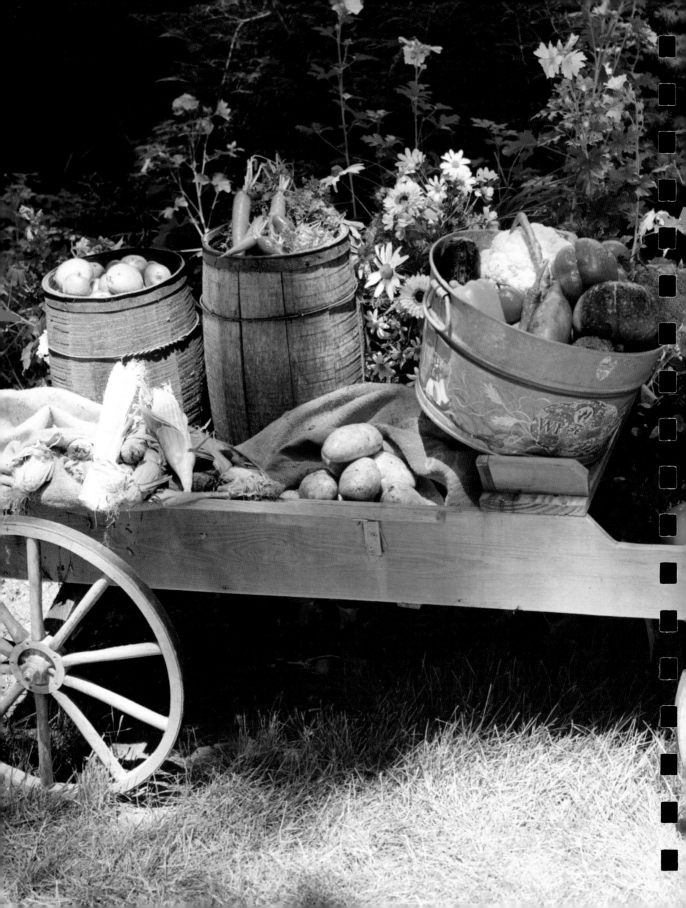

Chapter 1
VEGETABLE GROUP

Why eat vegetables?

Many studies have been done regarding vegetables and their health benefits. Among the discoveries are that vegetables are full of antioxidants and beta-carotene. They are believed to help us to resist diseases and some forms of cancer and coronary heart disease. Vegetables are high in vitamins A, B, C and valuable minerals and fiber.

And listen to this: Cruciferous vegetables such as broccoli and green leafy vegetables (spinach, mustard greens) seem to help lower the risk of ischemic strokes. Green leafy vegetables are also a good source of iron, essential for good red blood cells. Broccoli contains 200% of the RDA (Recommended Daily Allowance) of vitamin C. It's also full of vitamin A and fiber. And, vitamin A protects your eyesight. A vegetable's color also tells a story of its nutrition package. The brighter the color, especially red, orange and green, the more of a nutrition power-plant it is. (Ooh, a play on words!) But let's not forget our less flashy friends, like celery and potatoes. They are high in vitamin C and potassium! One medium potato contains 45% of vitamin C's RDA and 21% of the potassium recommended by the FDA. The skin of the potato is full of fiber, potassium, iron, calcium, zinc, phosphorus and B vitamins...so don't throw the skins away! See page 51 to find the wonderful recipe for baked potato skins inside this book. Great snack for watching the ballgames!

Let's get back to the vitamins: vitamin B is water soluble, so vegetables should be steamed or cooked in very little water. The more water in the pot, the more vitamins will be lost. But, steaming and cooking vegetables in the microwave will protect its nutritive value. They'll also stay firmer, and keep their color better. (don't you hate gray green beans?)

Good sources of vitamin C are tomatoes, green peppers, green leafy vegetables, celery, spinach, cabbage, potatoes. Vitamin C helps us to fight infections, prevents fatigue and promotes healing. Vitamin C, unlike vitamin A, cannot be stored up in the body so it has to be consumed every day. Good deal.

Tomatoes are naturally rich in the antioxidant lycopene, a relative of beta-carotene, which is a pigment predominantly found in tomatoes. It is believed to prevent certain kinds of cancer. Research has also found that processed tomato products (cooked sauces, tomato paste) contain 2–10 times as much lycopene as fresh tomatoes. Cooking tomatoes with olive oil helps us to absorb more lycopenes in our food, so cook 'em up! Delicious!

VEGETABLES: BUYING AND STORING TIPS

FRESH VEGETABLES: Look for in season bargains or grow your own, it's fun!

Acorn & Butternut Squash

Choose heavy, smooth, hard, deep yellow flesh squash. It should have dull, not shiny skin.

Storage: Store squash in a paper bag in the refrigerator or a cool dark place. Don't store in plastic, it traps the moisture. Squash will last for 2-3 months. Acorn squash will last 1-2 months. Hubbard squash will last 3-6 months.

Beets

Choose small, firm, smooth beets with thin roots. Cut green tops when putting beets away – they drain nutrition from the beet.

Storage: Refrigerate in perforated plastic bags. Beets will keep for up to 3 weeks.

Black Beans*

Beans are inexpensive, low-fat, easy to prepare and loaded with nutrients. Legumes are fiber rich and believed by some, to reduce the risk of some kinds of cancer. Soak beans overnight, and discard the water. They will be more digestible.

Storage: Store in tightly sealed containers at room temperature.

Broccoli*

Choose dark green broccoli with no yellow buds. Full of antioxidants, vitamins A, B & C, there is folic acid in the dark green leafy vegetables. Broccoli and broccoli sprouts are called the super vegetable, because they are so healthy and full of antioxidants.

Storage: Store in the vegetable crisper of the refrigerator.

Cabbage*

Excellent buy – choose cabbage that is heavy for its size. Leaves should be crisp and compact with no cracks or blemishes.

Storage: Store cabbage wrapped in a perforated plastic bag in the refrigerator.

Carrots

Look for firm and smooth carrots with no cracks. Color should be bright orange. They should not be limp and soft.

Storage: Store carrots for 2 weeks in an airtight container.

Cauliflower*

Buy creamy white cauliflower (no brown spots, they indicate bruising). It's believed that cauliflower reduces the risk of cancer. It's a great antioxidant.

Storage: Place in the vegetable drawer in the refrigerator.

*Cruciferae Family

Celery   Buy celery with firm stalks.

Storage: Store wrapped in aluminum foil in the refrigerator.

Chicory   Stems should be firm, crisp. They are from the same family as endive. The leaves should be red to purple, with no spots or blackened stems. Chicory is rich in calcium, phosphorous, vitamins B and C.

Storage: Store chicory in a cool place, like a refrigerator crisper.

Collard Greens*

Collards have a milder flavor than kale. There should be crisp, deep green leaves with no yellow tinge. Buy greens with smaller leaves.

Storage: Keeps in the refrigerator for 3 or 4 days.

Corn   When buying corn on the cob, the husk should be green and tight. The kernels should be plump and milky when pinched. If the kernels are large at the tip where the silk is located, they are over matured.

Storage: Fresh corn should be stored in a cool place. Warmth causes the sugar in the corn to turn to starch. This will make the corn less sweet, so cook the corn as soon as possible. Do not add salt when cooking, as it will toughen kernels.

Escarole   Buy crisp, firm packed heads of escarole. They have a milder flavor than endive.

Storage: Store in a plastic bag in the refrigerator.

Garlic   Buy firm, plump garlic bulbs with dry skin. Garlic is believed to reduce cholesterol.

Storage: Store in an open container in a cool dark place. Hanging bulbs in old panty hose will work. See storage for onions below. Plant garlic around rose bushes and it will repel bugs.

Green Peppers

Peppers should be firm and glossy, green stems, unwrinkled skin, bright color, no cracks. Colored peppers such as red, yellow, purple and orange are much more expensive than green peppers, but contain more vitamins.

Storage: Keep peppers in a plastic bag in the refrigerator.

Kale   Buy blue/green curly kale leaves that are not wilted. Avoid leaves that are getting yellow. Always tear the greens in salads. A knife will cause discoloration.

*Cruciferae Family

21

Storage: Place kale in a perforated (holes is bag) plastic bag in the refrigerator crisper. Use within a couple of days.

Mushrooms   Buy smooth, firm caps, free from blemishes, not shriveled or slimy.

Storage: Clean mushrooms with a damp cloth. Never soak mushrooms! They're like a sponge and will absorb water. Remove the store plastic wrap and cover with a white paper towel. You may also store mushrooms in a paper bag rather than plastic (moisture will build up in plastic).

Onion   Choose firm onions, with dry papery skin, and no spots or moisture. Onions should not smell.

In case you wondered why your eyes water when you are peeling them, it's because the sulfur combines with the water in your eyes causing irritation. Freeze the onion for 10 minutes to eliminate the problem. Also, cut the root end of the onion last.

Storage: Store onions in a cool dry place with good circulation. Onions will keep for 3 months. Hang them in the cellar. I use a nylon stocking and drop them in one at a time and tie a knot. I continue this until the nylon is full. This way, they get good circulation and can be cut off as needed.

Parsley   When buying parsley, look for firm stems, no blemishes, yellowing or wilting. Flat leaf parsley has more flavor and is used in cooking. Curly leaves are used more as a garnish. Parsley contains vitamin C. Chew on parsley after eating garlic and it will eliminate the smell and taste.

Storage: Wash, blot dry, and keep in a perforated plastic bag in the refrigerator.

Potatoes   Potatoes should have smooth skin with no sprouts. Russet is for baking, long and white is for boiling, round and white is for roasting, and round and red is for roasting and baking.

Storage: Store potatoes in a cool place away from onions, as they will cause them to rot. Place an apple in the bag and the potatoes will not sprout. Never store in the refrigerator, because the starch will turn to sugar. Potatoes keep well in burlap bags or brown bags with holes in them. Potatoes will keep for 2 months if stored properly. Don't store in foil. It seals in the moisture and causes soggy potatoes. Yuck!

Pumpkin*   Pumpkins should have no soft spots. They are rich in beta-carotene, and some are found to have scary faces carved into them at certain times of the year!

*Cruciferae Family

Storage: Store pumpkins at 50 to 55 degrees, on shelves, not a concrete floor in the cellar. There should be good circulation of air. Don't store near apples or other ripening fruits. Apples release ethylene gas causing a shortened storage life. Pumpkins will last for 2-3 months if properly stored – without the carved faces!

Romaine The lettuce should have dark green, crisp leaves, no rust spots or browning leaves. Romaine is a favorite when making Caesar salad.

Storage: Wash and dry romaine before storing. Separate leaves and place in a plastic bag in the refrigerator.

Rutabagas Rutabagas and turnips—how easy to mistake one for the other! Rutabagas are orange-yellow, while a turnip is white with a purple top. Rutabagas have a stronger flavor. Avoid buying if they look dry. (Not the weather; the rutabagas!)

Storage: Rutabagas keep well in the refrigerator for 10 days.

Spinach Spinach is always a good buy. Look for dark green unwilted leaves. Spinach is full of antioxidants and vitamins. Look what it did for Popeye...

Storage: Rinse and dry. Place spinach in covered container in the refrigerator.

String Beans Buy beans with vibrant green or yellow color, small in size that snap easily and are firm. There should be no bulge of bean in the shell. Bulging means the string bean is over mature. String beans will keep their color if you cook them uncovered.

Storage: Don't wash beans before storing, or it will cause brown spots. Store beans in a plastic bag in the refrigerator crisper.

Sweet Potatoes

Buy firm, smooth, thin-skinned potatoes with no cracks or bruises. They should have a sweet taste. Sweet potatoes are very high in beta-carotene. A real nutritional powerhouse here!

Storage: Place potatoes in a dry, cool place, not in the refrigerator.

Tomatoes Buy tomatoes that are bright red, plump, firm, and free from surface cracks and with no bruises.

*Cruciferae Family

Storage: Never refrigerate, it will spoil the texture, and diminish the nutritional value and taste. Think of cold, moist cardboard! Your taste buds deserve better! Room temperature tomatoes are happy tomatoes.

To prevent tomato stains in plastic containers, spray the container with cooking spray, before you add the tomato product.

Turnip   Purple top turnip (spring vegetable), has a milder flavor than rutabagas. It should have smooth, shiny, unwrinkled skin. Turnip also contains calcium and potassium.

Storage: Turnips keep well in the refrigerator for up to 10 days.

Yam   Yams have a tough, scaly skin and are long, cylindrical, dry and starchy. Yams are lower in beta-carotene then sweet potatoes.

Storage: Keep in a dry cool place.

FROZEN VEGETABLES

Wait for special sales. Buy vegetables in large plastic bags and divide up into daily portions. Frozen vegetables are processed and frozen at the peak of freshness. Packages of frozen vegetables should not be limp, sweating or wet. When you shake it, the vegetables should separate and not be in a frozen clump.

Storage: Store in the freezer.

CANNED VEGETABLES

When buying canned vegetables, make sure there are no leaks, large dents or bulges. All brands of canned vegetables contain the same food value. The only difference in brands is the flavor and eye appeal. How you plan on using the vegetable will determine what brand you should buy. Store brands are usually less expensive, and the larger cans are a better buy than the smaller ones. Try to buy in bulk, when canned vegetables go on sale. Cut and chopped vegetables cost less than whole. Buying cans with no salt is much healthier. If buying canned mushrooms, buy the stems and pieces. Many stores have canned vegetable sales – check the dates to make sure the can is not outdated. Canned vegetables are just as nutritious as frozen or fresh.

Storage: Canned vegetables can last as long as 5 years. Be sure to check the expiration date. Oldest cans should be placed in the front in your cabinet and the newest in the rear.

COOKING TECHNIQUES – VEGETABLES

FRESH

The food value received from vegetables is determined by the way it is cut and cooked. The more surface area exposed to air and water in cooking, the greater the loss of vitamins. When possible, leave skins on and cut vegetables, so there is little surface area exposed. Because vitamin B is water-soluble, you should cook vegetables with as little water as possible. Steaming is the best method. The kind of vegetable you are cooking will determine how much water you should use, and cook vegetables only until tender.

To retain the green color in your green vegetables, such as green beans and spinach, cook uncovered for the first few minutes, then cover.

The dark green outside leaves of cabbage and other green leafy vegetables are high in nutrition, so do not throw them away (unless they are very wilted). Use them for cabbage roll ups or in a New England boiled dinner.

Strong flavored vegetables, such as onions and turnips, may be cooked in a larger amount of water, if a milder flavor is desired.

Baking vegetables, such as potatoes, squash, turnips, etc., will also save on the food value.

FROZEN

Frozen vegetables are cooked according to the package directions. If using vegetables from large poly bags, be sure to use only the amount needed for your family. Tightly seal the remaining vegetables, in smaller freezer bags to prevent vitamin loss. Be sure to put the date on the vegetable freezer bags, and then you will know if they are outdated.

CANNED

Canned vegetables have already been cooked and only need to be heated. Heat canned vegetables as follows:

1. Pour juice of vegetable into saucepan.

2. Cook liquid until $1/2$ remains.

3. Add vegetable to hot liquid and cover. Take pan off heat and let vegetable heat in the liquid. Do not boil. Save any juice leftover from vegetables for soups and sauces.

NOTE: Americans' favorite vegetables are onions, tomatoes, and green beans. What are yours?

BAKED CABBAGE

Very inexpensive vegetable and so good for you.
My husband loves it with white vinegar.

To reduce cabbage odor when cooking, put a celery rib or lemon wedge into the pot.

Ingredients:
1 large head green cabbage
4 small red tomatoes, diced
1 small white onion, chopped
$\frac{1}{2}$ teaspoon garlic powder
$\frac{1}{2}$ teaspoon salt
1 teaspoon black pepper
$\frac{1}{8}$ cup water or chicken stock

Temp: 325°
Time: 30 minutes
Yields: 4-6 servings

Directions:
1. Quarter cabbage and boil in a large pot for 10 minutes.
2. Remove cabbage sections, place in shallow baking dish.
3. Combine other ingredients in a small bowl and pour over cabbage.
4. Bake.
5. Turn cabbage pieces halfway through cooking time so the topside does not overcook.

Crohn's Disease and IBS:
This recipe is not good for people with Crohn's, because cabbage is hard to digest and is very gassy.
Sugar 1 gm; **Fat** 2 gms

Diabetes:
Make your own chicken stock and skim off the fat. Enjoy!
Carbs 7 gms; **Calories** 33

Heart Disease:
Eliminate the salt and use your own chicken stock for this recipe. Cabbage is a cruciferous vegetable and full of antioxidants.
Sodium 22 mgs; **Cholesterol** 0 mgs

BAKED SUMMER SQUASH

Grated summer squash is a good substitute for carrots in carrot cake.

Add some of your favorite seasonings (lemon, dill, etc.) to steamed, sauteed, or grilled squash.

Ingredients:
1 medium squash
1 cup water
2 teaspoons brown sugar or Splenda brown sugar blend
2 teaspoons trans fat-free margarine or butter

Temp: 350°
Time: 30-60 minutes
Yields: 5-6 servings

Directions:
1. Cut off stem and blossom end of squash.
2. Cut in half, lengthwise.
3. Place squash into a glass baking dish.
4. Sprinkle with brown sugar and margarine.
5. Add a cup of water to the bottom of the baking dish.
6. Bake until tender.

Crohn's Disease and IBS:
Use light, trans fat-free margarine and Splenda.
Sugar 3 gms; **Fat** 2 gms

Diabetes:
Replace brown sugar with Splenda. The brown sugar in the recipe is only used as a sweetener.
Carbs 4 gms; **Calories** 18

Heart Disease:
Use a heart safe, light margarine in place of the butter.
Sodium 8 mgs; **Cholesterol** 0 mgs

BAKED WINTER SQUASH

Some of the winter squashes are acorn, butternut, and hubbard.
They are believed to help prevent macular degeneration.

Ingredients:
1 large acorn squash
Light butter or light, trans fat-free margarine
1 cup water
Salt and pepper to taste

Temp: 400°
Time: Acorn: 35 min per lb;
       Hubbard: 1 hour
Yields: 5-6 servings

Directions:
1. Take 3 pounds winter squash, wash and cut into individual servings.
2. Remove seeds and stringy parts.
3. Season with salt, pepper, and butter or margarine. Add water.
4. Place in a large baking pan.
5. Bake uncovered for crusty top; covered for a moist top.
6. Baking squash without peeling will save on the food value.

Crohn's Disease and IBS:
Use light, trans fat-free margarine.
Sugar 1 gm; **Fat** 5 gms

Diabetes:
Eliminate the salt and enjoy! Use a light, trans fat-free margarine with 0 carbs.
Carbs 30 gms; **Calories** 160

Heart Disease:
Eliminate the salt and use heart-safe, light margarine. Enjoy!
Sodium 8 mgs; **Cholesterol** 0 mgs

BOILED ONIONS

Cooking onions will turn the sulfur into sugar, that's why onions are sweeter when cooked. It's the sulfur that makes eyes water. Freeze for 10 minutes before peeling and cutting.

Onions should never be stored near potatoes. They release gases that will alter the taste of potatoes.

Ingredients:
15 small white onions
Salt and pepper to taste
Water
Light butter or trans fat-free margarine

Temp: Medium heat
Time: 20-30 minutes
Yields: 4 servings

Directions:
1. To avoid irritation to eyes when peeling onions, place them in the freezer for 10 or 15 minutes. This will harden the juices inside the onion.
2. Peel.
3. To keep the center of the onion from popping out, puncture it with a sharp object – large needle, etc.
4. Place onions in a saucepan with a lot of water for a milder flavor or a little water for a stronger flavor.
5. Cook onions about 25 to 30 minutes, depending on the size.
6. Serve with salt, pepper, and butter or margarine.

Crohn's Disease and IBS:
Use a light margarine spray instead of the butter. Onions may cause stomach upset, eat in moderation. I usually cook onions a little longer in fresh water.
Sugar 2 gms; **Fat** 1 gm

Diabetes:
Use a light margarine spray.
Carbs 7 gms; **Calories** 32

Heart Disease:
Eliminate salt and use a light margarine spray. Read the label.
Sodium 3 mgs; **Cholesterol** 0 mgs

BOILED TURNIP (White)

Yellow rutabagas have a stronger flavor than purple top turnip,
so cook it in more water. They also take longer to cook.

Ingredients:
1 purple top turnip
Water
Salt and pepper to taste
Light, trans fat-free spray
Trans fat-free margarine

Temp: Medium heat
Time: 15-30 minutes
Yields: 4-5 servings

Directions:
1. Scrub, but do not peel. (Helps to retain vitamins and food value.)
2. Cut into large pieces.
3. Cook in a covered saucepan in a small amount of water for 15 to 30 minutes.
4. Remove from pan. Peel and mash.
5. Season with salt, pepper, and light butter or trans fat-free margarine.

Crohn's Disease and IBS:
Turnip will be hard for Crohn's people to digest. Not recommended. If you do eat it, use a light margarine spray.
Sugar 2 gms; **Fat** 2 gms

Diabetes:
Use a light margarine spray.
Carbs 8 gms; **Calories** 48

Heart Disease:
Eliminate the salt. Spices may be used in place of salt (example: garlic powder). Use a light margarine spray.
Sodium 23 mgs; **Cholesterol** 0 mgs

BROCCOLI CASSEROLE

According to the USDA, broccoli contains more vitamin C than an orange, and as much fiber as a slice of whole grain bread.

Ingredients:
2 bunches fresh or frozen broccoli florets
2 tablespoons trans fat-free margarine or butter
2 tablespoons all-purpose, unbleached flour (organic)
1 cup low-fat milk
Salt and pepper to taste
$\frac{1}{2}$ a low-sodium chicken bouillon cube or your own chicken stock
1 small bag seasoned stuffing mix
$\frac{1}{4}$ cup butter or trans fat-free margarine
$\frac{1}{2}$ cup water

Temp: 350°
Time: 30 minutes
Yields: 6 servings

Directions:
1. Cook the broccoli in a steamer until fork tender.
2. Place into the bottom of a 9x12 greased casserole dish.
3. Make a medium white sauce by melting 2 tablespoons butter or trans fat-free margarine over medium to low heat. Add 2 tablespoons flour and $\frac{1}{2}$ a chicken bouillon cube. Stir to make a paste.
4. Add 1 cup milk and stir over low heat until it thickens.
5. Pour white sauce over broccoli.
6. Melt remaining butter in a frying pan.
7. Add the water and seasoned crumbs and lightly brown.
8. Place seasoned crumbs on top of the white sauce and broccoli.
9. Bake.

Crohn's Disease and IBS:
Change the low-fat milk to either soy or nondairy milk. Butter should be eliminated. Use a light, trans fat-free margarine, or light spray.
Sugar 2 gms; **Fat** 4 gms

Diabetes:
Use gluten-free flour and crumbs. Use a light spray in place of margarine as there are no carbs and calories. Substitute fat-free skim milk for the low-fat milk.
Carbs 12 gms; **Calories** 46

Heart Disease:
Eliminate the salt and use your own chicken stock. Chicken bouillon cubes are high in sodium. Replace the butter with a heart-safe, light margarine. Read the label to select the best. Use a light spray. It contains no sodium or cholesterol. The sodium is located in the seasoned crumbs. Look for low-sodium crumbs.
Sodium 57 mgs; **Cholesterol** 0 mgs

BROCCOLI SAUTÉ

We should all get rid of our salt shakers and only use spices for flavor.

Ingredients:
2 pounds fresh broccoli (4 stalks)
$1/2$ cup water
$1/4$ cup canola oil
2 cloves minced garlic
1 teaspoon Mrs. Dash (no salt spices)
$1/8$ teaspoon pepper

Temp: Medium heat
Time: 20-30 minutes
Yields: 4 servings

Directions:
1. Clean broccoli and cut into large stalks.
2. Place in a large saucepan.
3. Sprinkle with water, oil, garlic, Mrs. Dash, and pepper.
4. Cover and simmer over medium heat for 20-30 minutes.

Crohn's Disease and IBS:
Broccoli can be gassy, but I have found that the benefits are worth it.
Sugar 1 gm; **Fat** 2 gms

Diabetes:
This recipe is fine for diabetics. Eliminate the salt and use a salt substitute. Enjoy!
Carbs 10 gms; **Calories** 54

Heart Disease:
Eliminate the salt and use a salt substitute. Enjoy!
Sodium 48 mgs; **Cholesterol** 0 mgs

DRAKE'S COLESLAW

As a child we would have this coleslaw every Saturday night with homemade baked beans.

Mel Blanc, the voice of Bugs Bunny, didn't like carrots!

Ingredients:
1 head cabbage
3 large carrots
1 (20-ounce) can sugar-free crushed pineapple
Reduced-fat mayonnaise or plain low-fat yogurt to taste*

Time: 10 minutes
Yields: 6 servings

Read the label on low-fat foods, make sure they didn't add extra sugar to make up for the lost fat.

Directions:
1. Using grater, shred cabbage and carrots.
2. Add crushed pineapple.
3. Mix enough mayonnaise to suit your taste.

Crohn's Disease and IBS:
Not recommended.
Sugar 2 gms; **Fat** 2 gms

Diabetes:
Mix the coleslaw with yogurt instead of mayonnaise. Or use the Estee lower calorie mayonnaise (contains only 61 calories).
Carbs 14 gms; **Calories** 83

Heart Disease:
Use Estee lower calorie mayonnaise (contains only 3 mgs of sodium).
Sodium 42 mgs; **Cholesterol** 0 mgs

SAUTÉED COLLARDS AND KALE

Greens are very high in antioxidants,
believed to protect your eyes from macular degeneration.

Don't burn the garlic; it will taste bitter! Garlic is a wonderful antioxidant.

Ingredients:
1 large bunch collards
1 large bunch kale
Canola oil (can cook at a higher heat)
6 cloves garlic, finely chopped
1/4 teaspoon salt or Mrs. Dash
1/2 teaspoon pepper
4 teaspoons lemon juice

Temp: Medium to medium-high
Time: Until tender
Yields: 4+ servings

Directions:
1. Rinse collards and kale in a large bowl of water.
2. Drain and cut off the tough stems.
3. There should be approximately 3/4 pound of each green.
4. Cut leaves into 1/4 inch strips.
5. There should be 6-8 tightly packed cups.
6. In a well-seasoned heavy pan or wok, heat the oil in moderate to high heat.
7. Add the chopped garlic and cook about 30 seconds.
8. Next, add approximately 1/2 of the greens and cook another 30 seconds.
9. Add the second 1/2 of the greens and cook until they begin to wilt.
10. Cook, stirring constantly, for approximately 8 minutes.
11. Greens will darken and become tender.
12. Season with salt, pepper and lemon juice.

Crohn's Disease and IBS:
Cut greens well and cook until tender using a light cooking spray. Cook garlic whole and take out of pan when done.
Sugar 2 gms; **Fat** 3 gms

Diabetes:
Do not add salt and cook in a light cooking spray.
Carbs 17 gms; **Calories** 85

Heart Disease:
Do not add salt and use a light cooking spray.
Sodium 50 mgs; **Cholesterol** 0 gms

FALL VEGETABLE MEDLEY

Rutabaga is a yellow winter turnip and has a very strong flavor.
It's stronger than the spring purple top turnip.

Ingredients:
½ pound rutabaga peeled and cut in julienne strips
1 parsnip peeled and sliced into round cubes
1 small zucchini cut into julienne strips
2 carrots, peeled and cut into julienne strips
1 tablespoon extra virgin olive oil or light spray
Pepper to taste

Temp: Medium
Time: 10 minutes
Yields: 6 servings

Directions:
1. Steam vegetables until tender, about 10 minutes.
2. Warm the olive oil in a skillet (don't let it sizzle).
3. Add the vegetables and toss, so they are coated with the oil.
4. When the edges of the vegetables start to brown, remove from oil.
5. Sprinkle with pepper and serve.

Crohn's Disease and IBS:
Not recommended.
Sugar 2 gms; **Fat** 3 gms

Diabetes:
Just steam the vegetables and put them under the broiler to brown.
Carbs 5 gms; **Calories** 25

Heart Disease:
Just steam the vegetables and put them under the broiler to brown.
Sodium 10 mgs; **Cholesterol** 0 mgs

GARLIC POTATOES

Small red potatoes work very well in this dish.

Ingredients:
1 pound small potatoes (approximately 3 medium size)
1 teaspoon extra virgin olive oil or light spray
4 cloves garlic, peeled and thickly sliced
1 tablespoon minced shallots
1/8 teaspoon salt
Pepper to taste
1 teaspoon chopped parsley

Temp: 350°
Time: 30 minutes
Yields: 4 servings

Directions:
1. Scrub potatoes.
2. Cut into 4-6 pieces.
3. Steam for 7 minutes until firm, but slightly tender.
4. Pour oil into a 9x5x3 casserole dish.
5. Add the steamed potatoes, garlic slices, shallots, salt, and pepper.
6. Toss and mix well.
7. Bake uncovered. Stir a few times to insure even cooking.
8. Sprinkle with parsley.

Crohn's Disease and IBS:
Use garlic powder in place of the garlic.
Sugar 1 gm; **Fat** 3 gms

Diabetes:
Fine to eat.
Carbs 20 gms; **Calories** 86

Heart Disease:
Just eliminate the salt and enjoy.
Sodium trace; **Cholesterol** 0 mgs

ORIGINAL GREEN BEAN CASSEROLE

As kids, while living in Maine, we went bean picking during the summer months. We would earn 12 cents a bushel, enough to pay for school supplies.

Ingredients:
³/₄ cup low-fat milk
1 (10 ³/₄-ounce) can low-sodium cream of mushroom soup
2 (15¹/₄-ounce) cans low-salt drained green beans
1¹/₃ cup French fried onions (You know, the kind in the can!)
¹/₈ teaspoon pepper

Temp: 350°
Time: 35 minutes
Yields: 6 servings

Directions:
1. Mix all the ingredients except ¹/₂ cup of fried onions.
2. Place in a 1¹/₂ quart casserole dish.
3. Bake 30 minutes and stir.
4. Top with remaining onions and bake for another 5 minutes.

Crohn's Disease and IBS:
Use French style green beans… the fiber has been cut and they are easier to digest. Also use a nondairy milk and a low-fat cream of mushroom soup. I sometimes make a medium white sauce (found on page 31) and add mushrooms instead of soup.
Sugar 2 gms; **Fat** 3.5 gms

Diabetes:
Use nonfat skim milk. Slice sweet onions and use those instead of the French fried onion rings.
Carbs 16 gms; **Calories** 54

Heart Disease:
Use nonfat skim milk. Slice onion and use those instead of the French fried onions. Use no salt added green beans.
Sodium 10 mgs; **Cholesterol** 0 mgs

KALE

Ingredients:
1 pound kale
1 cup water
$\frac{1}{2}$ teaspoon salt
2 tablespoons butter or trans fat-free margarine
1 hard cooked egg

Temp: Medium heat
Time: 15-20 minutes
Yields: 4-5 servings

Directions:
1. Cut off root and wash kale thoroughly.
2. Remove heavy stems from leaves.
3. Place kale in saucepan containing 1 cup water.
4. Cover and cook 15 to 20 minutes.
5. Drain, chop, and add butter or margarine and salt to the cooked kale.
6. Sprinkle the top with the chopped egg.

Crohn's Disease and IBS:
If you want to eat the kale, make sure you cook it very thoroughly. I have found if I cut against the fibers I have less trouble eating kale, lettuce, etc. Only use the white of the hard cooked egg.
Sugar 2 gms; **Fat** 2 gms

Diabetes:
Use trans fat-free or Smart Balance margarine in place of the butter. Use only the whites of the chopped egg.
Carbs 7 gms; **Calories** 12

Heart Disease:
Eliminate the salt and only use the white of the chopped egg. Use the trans fat-free margarine.
Sodium 40 mgs; **Cholesterol** 0 mgs

SCALLOPED POTATOES

The average American eats 124 pounds of potatoes every year.
Germans eat twice as much.

Ingredients:
6 medium potatoes
3 tablespoons butter or trans fat-free margarine
2½ tablespoons all-purpose, unbleached flour (organic)
3 cups low-fat milk
1 teaspoon salt
¼ teaspoon pepper
1 chopped onion (Put onion in freezer 10-15 minutes before chopping to harden juices. This will eliminate eye irritation.)

Temp: 350°
Time: 1 hour
Yields: 4-6 servings

Directions:
1. Peel potatoes and slice thin. Use a potato peeler to get real thin slices.
2. Melt margarine in saucepan; blend in flour, salt, pepper and milk.
3. Cook over medium heat until thickened, stirring constantly.
4. Alternate layers of potato, onions, and sauce in a greased 2-quart casserole.
5. Top with remaining sauce.
6. Cover and bake.
7. Uncover for the last 10 minutes to allow top to brown.

Crohn's Disease and IBS:
Use nondairy milk and light, trans fat-free margarine.
Sugar 1 gm; **Fat** 3 gms

Diabetes:
Replace a light, trans fat-free margarine for the butter. Use gluten-free flour and no salt.
Carbs 18 gms; **Calories** 84

Heart Disease:
Use a trans fat-free margarine and skim milk. Eliminate the salt.
Sodium 7 mgs; **Cholesterol** 0 mgs

SLICED BAKED POTATOES

Ingredients:
4 medium potatoes (I use Idaho.)
½ teaspoon salt
2 to 3 tablespoons melted butter or trans fat-free margarine
2 to 3 tablespoons mixed herbs (parsley, thyme, and chives - Mrs. Dash seasoning is good*)
2 tablespoons herb of your choice
4 tablespoons Alpine Lace nonfat cheddar cheese
1½ tablespoons low-fat Parmesan cheese

Mrs. Dash seasoning is all natural and contains no salt.

Temp: 425°
Time: 50 minutes
Yields: 4 servings

Directions:
1. Peel potatoes or scrub clean and rinse.
2. Cut potatoes into thin slices approximately ⅔ through.
3. Put potatoes in a baking dish. Fan them slightly.
4. Sprinkle with salt, drizzle with butter and sprinkle with herbs.
5. Bake about 35 to 40 minutes.
6. Remove from oven and sprinkle with cheese.
7. Bake potatoes for another 10-15 minutes until lightly browned.
8. Check with fork for tenderness.

Crohn's Disease and IBS:
Substitute a light, trans fat-free margarine for the butter. Use a nondairy cheese in place of the cheddar and Parmesan. Soy cheese is delicious.
Sugar 2 gms; **Fat** 3 gms

Diabetes:
Use low-fat cheese and a light, trans fat-free margarine in place of the cheeses and butter. Eliminate the salt and use a salt substitute.
Carbs 18 gms; **Calories** 122

Heart Disease:
Use a light, trans fat-free margarine in place of the butter. Eliminate the salt and use a salt substitute.
Sodium 70 mgs; **Cholesterol** 0 mgs

STEAMED WINTER SQUASH

Ingredients:
1 large butternut squash
Butter or trans fat-free margarine
Salt and pepper to taste
Pinch of cinnamon, optional

Temp: Medium to medium-high heat
Time: 40-45 minutes
Yields: 3-4 servings

Directions:
1. Cut squash into pieces, removing the seeds and stringy parts.
2. Leave the peelings on to prevent vitamin loss.
3. Steam over boiling water until tender.
4. Cook about 40-45 minutes.
5. Remove from pan. Peel, cool, and mash.
6. Season with salt, pepper, and margarine.

Crohn's Disease and IBS:
Substitute the butter with a light, trans fat-free margarine. Use cinnamon in place of salt.
Sugar 1 gm; **Fat** 3 gms

Diabetes:
Replace the butter with a light, trans fat-free margarine. Use cinnamon in place of salt.
Carbs 4 gms; **Calories** 16

Heart Disease:
Use a light, trans fat-free margarine and no salt. Use cinnamon instead of salt.
Sodium Trace; **Cholesterol** 0 mgs

STUFFED GREEN PEPPERS

Ingredients:
6 large green peppers
$1/2$ pound lean hamburger (93% fat-free, plus 1 tablespoon of canola oil to make it moist)
$1/2$ pound all white meat ground turkey
2 tablespoons chopped onions
1 teaspoon salt
$1/8$ teaspoon chopped garlic
1 cup cooked rice (brown rice)
1 (15-ounce) can tomato sauce
$3/4$ cup shredded low-fat mozzarella cheese

Temp: 350°
Time: 60 minutes
Yields: 6 servings

Directions:
1. Prepare pepper by removing a thin slice from the stem end of the pepper.
2. Take seeds and membranes out of peppers.
3. Rinse inside of the peppers.
4. Place peppers in boiling water for 5 minutes.
5. Drain.
6. In a 10-inch skillet, cook onions, garlic, hamburger and/or ground turkey.
7. Stir in salt, cooked rice and 1 cup of tomato sauce.
8. Stand peppers upright in a greased 8x8 casserole dish.
9. Cover with remaining tomato sauce.
10. Cover and cook for 45 minutes.
11. Uncover and bake for 15 minutes more.
12. Sprinkle with mozzarella and place back in the oven until the cheese is melted.
13. Serve warm.

Crohn's Disease and IBS:
Cook green pepper and onions an additional 3 minutes. They will be easier to digest. Use a nondairy cheese such as soy cheese. Use only ground turkey.
Sugar 3 gms; **Fat** 5 gms

Diabetes:
Use gluten-free rice found in the health food stores. Some grocery stores are selling gluten-free products. Use only ground turkey.
Carbs 19 gms; **Calories** 121

Heart Disease:
Use only a pound of ground turkey, no beef. Eliminate the salt. Replace the tomato sauce with salt-free sauce.
Sodium 31 mgs; **Cholesterol** 17 mgs

SWEET POTATO CASSEROLE

My daughter makes this dish for our Thanksgiving meal every year.
Never put sweet potatoes in your refrigerator unless they have been cooked,
they will spoil much faster. Keep at room temperature.

Ingredients:
3 cups cooked mashed sweet potatoes
$^3/_4$ cup white sugar or Splenda
2 eggs or egg substitute
Dash of cinnamon
$^3/_4$ cup trans fat-free margarine
1 can low-fat condensed milk

Temp: 400°
Time: 35 minutes
Yields: 6 servings

Directions:
1. Mix all ingredients until well blended.
2. Pour into a buttered baking dish.
3. Bake.

Crumb Topping:
1 cup crushed corn flakes (organic corn flakes have less sodium)
1 cup chopped pecans or walnuts
$^1/_2$ cup brown sugar or Splenda brown sugar blend
$^1/_2$ cup butter or trans fat-free margarine

Directions:
1. Melt margarine and stir in remaining ingredients.
2. Sprinkle on the top of potatoes.
3. Bake for an additional 15 minutes.

Crohn's Disease and IBS:
Change sugar to Splenda, milk to nondairy milk (soy) and butter to a light, trans fat-free margarine. Use egg substitute.
Sugar 4 gms; **Fat** 20 gms

Diabetes:
Change sugar to Splenda, milk to skim milk, corn flakes to gluten free flakes, and butter to trans fat-free margarine.
Carbs 20 gms; **Calories** 96

Heart Disease:
Replace the whole eggs with egg substitute or 4 egg whites. Replace butter with a heart-safe margarine. Use organic corn flakes.
Sodium 74 mgs; **Cholesterol** Trace

TWICE BAKED POTATOES

Potatoes are full of potassium, 750 mg in one medium potato. Don't refrigerate or wash before storing. Washing speeds decay. Baking potatoes instead of boiling will retain more nutrients. Avoid green potatoes. They have been exposed to too much light and have a bitter taste.

Ingredients:
6 medium baking potatoes
Salt and pepper to taste
Low-fat milk, 1 teaspoon per potato
Butter or trans fat-free margarine
Toppings (broccoli, cheese, paprika, bacon bits, etc.)

Temp: 425°
Time: 1 hour
Yields: 6 servings

Directions:
1. Rub potatoes with a little butter or margarine.
2. Bake until potatoes are soft when pressed.
3. Slash potato skins lengthwise.
4. Fold back flaps; scoop out inside and whip with salt, pepper, milk, and butter or margarine.
5. Place whipped potatoes back in the shell, sprinkle with paprika, bacon bits, broccoli, and cheese. (select desired toppings)
6. Bake in oven until potatoes are brown on top.

Crohn's Disease and IBS:
Use nondairy milk, soy cheese, and light, trans fat-free margarine. Eliminate bacon.
Sugar 5 gms; **Fat** 4 gms

Diabetes:
Use skim milk, no bacon, and trans fat-free margarine.
Carbs 17 gms; **Calories** 82

Heart Disease:
Eliminate salt, bacon, and use low-fat cheese, and skim milk.
Sodium 14 mgs; **Cholesterol** 2 mgs

ANDY'S VEGETABLE FOIL PACKETS

Ingredients:
2 medium potatoes
2 carrots
1 medium sweet onion
1 green bell pepper
Heavy duty aluminum foil
Extra virgin olive oil
Butter or trans fat-free margarine or cooking spray
Salt and pepper to taste

Temp: Medium heat
Time: About 35 minutes
Yields: 2 servings

Directions:
1. Peel and cut potatoes into bite size pieces.
2. Cut carrots, onions, and pepper into bite size pieces.
3. Place above ingredients onto double layer or heavy-duty aluminum foil (18″ by approximately 20″ long).
4. Add olive oil, butter or margarine, salt and pepper, and seal packet.
5. Grill until tender over medium heat.
6. For more servings, prepare additional packets.
7. Use caution when opening packets, as they will be hot.

Crohn's Disease and IBS:
Use trans fat-free margarine.
Sugar 3 gms; **Fat** 5 gms

Diabetes:
Use trans fat-free margarine.
Carbs 14 gms; **Calories** 61

Heart Disease:
Eliminate the salt and use a heart-safe margarine.
Sodium 16 mgs; **Cholesterol** 0 mgs

VEGETARIAN LASAGNA

My sister, Jacqui, makes this vegetable lasagna for my Dad's Christmas party every year...it's a big hit with crowds.

Ingredients:
$^1/_2$ cup chopped onion
$^1/_4$ cup chopped celery
1 clove garlic, crushed
2 tablespoons vegetable oil (canola)
$1^1/_2$ cups mushrooms, sliced
1 (14-ounce) can tomato sauce
1 ($5^1/_2$-ounce) can tomato paste
1 teaspoon salt
1 carrot (as a sweetener)
$^1/_2$ teaspoon oregano
$^1/_4$ teaspoon each of pepper, thyme, and basil
6-8 lasagna noodles, cooked (whole grain)
$^1/_2$ pound low-fat ricotta or dry, low-fat cottage cheese
1 egg or 2 egg whites
2 tablespoons chopped parsley
$^1/_2$ teaspoon salt (2nd amount)
2 cups chopped, cooked spinach
1 cup sliced, cooked zucchini
1 cup sliced, cooked onions
8-ounces low-fat mozzarella, sliced
$^1/_4$ cup grated low-fat Parmesan cheese

Temp: 350°
Time: 30-40 minutes
Yields: 8 servings

continued on next page

Directions:
1. Cook onions, celery, and garlic in olive oil.
2. Add mushrooms, tomato sauce, tomato paste.
3. Mix salt, oregano, pepper, thyme and basil and add to the sauce.
4. Simmer sauce over medium heat, for 10 minutes.
5. Use a wooden spoon to stir the sauce. (won't conduct heat)
6. In a small mixing bowl, combine ricotta cheese with egg, parsley and 1/2 teaspoon salt.
7. Spread 1/2 cup tomato sauce mixture on the bottom of a 9x13 inch pan.
8. Arrange 1/2 the cooked noodles over sauce.
9. Put 1/2 the ricotta mixture over noodles, then half the well drained spinach, zucchini, and sliced onions.
10. Then 1/2 the tomato sauce mixture, 1/2 the mozzarella.
11. Repeat from the noodle layer.
12. Sprinkle with Parmesan cheese.
13. Bake.
14. Let stand for a few minutes before cutting.

Crohn's Disease and IBS:
Always substitute nondairy cheese and dairy products. I have Crohn's disease and make a small, nondairy lasagna for me, and the regular lasagna for my family. Soy cheese works for me.
Sugar 2 gms; **Fat** 6 gms

Diabetes:
Use gluten-free lasagna. Gluten-free products are now available at most grocery stores. Use low-fat cheeses.
Carbs 45 gms; **Calories** 114

Heart Disease:
Use 2 egg whites in place of the whole egg. Substitute low-fat cheese for ricotta and mozzarella. Be sure to eliminate the salt. If you are on a blood thinner, avoid spinach, as it contains vitamin K (promotes blood clotting).
Sodium 120 mgs; **Cholesterol** 25 mgs

GRILLED CORN ON THE COB

Ingredients:
4 ears of fresh corn with silks and husk
Butter or trans fat-free margarine
Salt and pepper to taste

Temp: Hot grill
Time: Until tender
Yields: 4 servings

Directions:
1. Soak corn in water for 30 minutes.
2. Remove corn from water and pull down husk and remove silk. Fold husk back in place.
3. Arrange corn on grill. Close lid of grill.
4. Cook, turning frequently until corn is fork tender.
5. Cool slightly and remove husk.
6. Brush with butter or trans fat-free margarine.
7. Sprinkle with salt and pepper to taste... easy on the salt!

Crohn's Disease and IBS:
Not recommended.
Sugar 2 gms; **Fat** .09 gms

Diabetes:
There is sugar in corn.
Carbs 14 gms; **Calories** 63

Heart Disease:
Eliminate the salt.
Sodium 13 mgs; **Cholesterol** 0 mgs

ZUCCHINI PARMESAN

Ingredients:
¼ cup extra virgin olive oil
8 medium zucchini, thinly sliced
⅓ cup coarsely chopped onions
2 tablespoons chopped parsley
1 large clove garlic, minced
Salt to taste
¼ teaspoon pepper
¼ teaspoon oregano
4 cups peeled chopped tomatoes
½ cup grated low fat Parmesan cheese

Temp: Medium heat
Time: 25 minutes
Yields: 8-10 servings

Directions:
1. Heat oil in large pan.
2. Add zucchini, onion, parsley, garlic, salt, pepper, and oregano.
3. Sauté over medium heat, stirring until zucchini is tender (approx. 20 minutes).
4. Add the chopped tomatoes.
5. Place on a serving platter and sprinkle with Parmesan cheese.

Crohn's Disease and IBS:
Use a nondairy Parmesan cheese in place of the grated Parmesan. Also be sure to peel the zucchini as the skin will be hard to digest.
Sugar 1 gm; **Fat** 6 gms

Diabetes:
Always use a low-fat grated Parmesan cheese. Eliminate the salt.
Carbs 5 gms; **Calories** 62

Heart Disease:
Eliminate the salt in all recipes and use low-fat cheeses.
Sodium 130 mgs; **Cholesterol** 0 mgs

MRS. CARRIER'S EGGPLANT PARMESAN

Ingredients:
2 small or one large eggplant
2 tablespoons extra virgin olive oil
2 eggs or 4 egg whites
¼ cup 1% milk
1½ cups seasoned bread crumbs…more, if needed* (crumbs should have no MSG)
1 cup all-purpose, unbleached flour (organic)
Pepper to taste
¼ cup parsley
1 (29-ounce) can tomato sauce
Canola oil
1 carrot (for sweetness)
½ teaspoon each oregano and sweet basil
1 clove fresh crushed garlic
1 cup grated low fat Parmesan cheese…more, if needed

Temp: 350°
Time: 30 minutes
Yields: 6 servings

To make breadcrumbs, toast a low-salt bread and place it in the blender. Blend with some parsley and spices. Store in covered jar. (also see page 102)

Directions:
1. Peel and thinly slice the eggplant.
2. Mix the eggs and milk in a medium bowl…set aside for later.
3. Combine the crumbs and flour in a shallow dish…set aside for later.
4. Dip the sliced eggplant in the egg mixture, then the flour mixture.
5. Cook eggplant in a frying pan, in the olive or vegetable oil, until lightly browned.
6. Blot the cooked eggplant on paper towels.
7. In a medium saucepan, make your favorite tomato sauce.
8. Cook garlic, oregano, and sweet basil in canola oil.
9. Add a teaspoon of brown sugar or a carrot.
10. In a 13x9 casserole dish start layering sauce, cooked eggplant, and Parmesan cheese. End with the cheese.
11. Bake covered.

Crohn's Disease and IBS:
Substitute dairy products with a nondairy milk and cheese. Use egg substitute.
Sugar 3 gms; **Fat** 5 gms

Diabetes:
Use gluten-free unseasoned breadcrumbs and flour.
Carbs 19 gms; **Calories** 149

Heart Disease:
Use only egg whites or egg substitute to dip eggplant into. Use homemade breadcrumbs, most crumbs contain too much sodium.*
Sodium 75 mgs; **Cholesterol** 1 mg

POTATO SKINS

Great treat for watching ballgames.

Ingredients:
4 russet potatoes (thick skinned potatoes)
¼ teaspoon black pepper
1 tablespoon chives
Salt to taste (I use a pepper mill to grind the salt)
Cooking spray
1 cup low-fat shredded cheddar cheese
Low-fat sour cream

Temp: 400°
Time: 1 hour
Yields: 6 servings

Directions:
1. Preheat oven to 400°.
2. Scrub potatoes and remove any blemishes with a paring knife.
3. Pat dry. Wrap individually in aluminum foil and bake.
4. Remove from the oven and unwrap. Be sure to wear oven mitts.
5. Let stand for 5 to 10 minutes. Cut each in half, lengthwise.
6. Gently scrape the inside of the potato out, but not all the way to the skin.
7. Leave an amount of the white flesh next to the skin.
8. Refrigerate potato scoopings for use in another recipe. (example, Swedish meatballs – see page 125)
9. Spray a large pan with the cooking spray and place the skins white side up.
10. Sprinkle the skins with the salt and pepper, and cooking spray or melted butter.
11. Broil skins for 6 to 8 minutes.
12. Sprinkle 2 to 3 tablespoons of cheese into each skin.
13. Broil the skins for 2 more minutes, or until the cheese is melted.
14. Mix the sour cream and chives.
15. Serve hot with the sour cream and chive dip.

Crohn's Disease and IBS:
Use a nondairy cheese and sour cream.
Sugar 9 gms; **Fat** 5 gms

Diabetes:
Replace cheese with only 1 cup of a fat-free cheddar cheese.
Carbs 6 gms; **Calories** 102

Heart Disease:
Eliminate the salt. Use Alpine Lace low-sodium cheese.
Sodium 10 mgs; **Cholesterol** 28 mgs

BETTE'S HOMEMADE THOUSAND ISLAND DRESSING

Ingredients: **Yields:** 2 cups

1¼ cup mayonnaise (low-fat, made with canola oil) or plain yogurt
²/₃ cup chili sauce
1½ tablespoons sweet pickle relish
1 egg yolk
1 teaspoon vinegar

Directions:
1. Mix all the above ingredients together.
2. Store in a tightly covered container in refrigerator.

Crohn's Disease and IBS:
Don't eat chili sauce unless you can tolerate it.
Sugar 3 gms; **Fat** 4 gms

Diabetes:
Use low-fat yogurt and only ½ tablespoon of the relish. Weight Watchers light mayonnaise has less carbs and calories.
Carbs 1 gm; **Calories** 19

Heart Disease:
Replace the whole eggs with egg substitute.
Sodium 63 mgs; **Cholesterol** 25 mgs

EVAPORATED MILK DRESSING

Ingredients:

Yields: 1⅓ cups

½ cup sugar or Splenda
⅓ cup vinegar
½ cup low-fat evaporated milk
½ teaspoon salt

Directions:
1. Add sugar to vinegar.
2. Stir until sugar is dissolved.
3. Beat in milk until mixture thickens.
4. Add salt.
5. Store in covered bottle in refrigerator.

Crohn's Disease and IBS:
Replace the evaporated milk with nondairy milk. Use Splenda.
Sugar 2 gms; **Fat** 3 gms

Diabetes:
Use Splenda in place of sugar. It's only as a sweetener.
Carbs 4 gms; **Calories** 20

Heart Disease:
Eliminate the salt. Use Splenda.
Sodium 21 mgs; **Cholesterol** 1 mg

ITALIAN DRESSING

Ingredients:

Yields: ³/₄ cup

1 clove garlic
¹/₂ teaspoon dried mustard
¹/₂ teaspoon salt
4 tablespoons red wine vinegar
¹/₂ cup extra virgin olive oil

Directions:
1. Peel and crush a clove of garlic.
2. Mix mustard, salt, garlic, and vinegar thoroughly.
3. Add oil and stir until all ingredients are blended.
4. Store in covered jar in refrigerator.
5. Shake well before using.

Crohn's Disease and IBS:
Eat in moderation.
Sugar 2 gms; **Fat** 7 gms

Diabetes:
Eliminate the salt or use a salt substitute.
Carbs 8 gms; **Calories** 4

Heart Disease:
Eliminate the salt or use a salt substitute.
Sodium 2 mgs; **Cholesterol** 0 mgs

FRENCH DRESSING

Ingredients: **Yields:** $^3/_4$-1 cup
$^1/_4$ to $^1/_2$ cup vinegar
$^1/_2$ cup canola or vegetable oil
1 teaspoon sugar or Splenda
$^1/_2$ teaspoon dry mustard
Dash of pepper
1 teaspoon paprika
1 clove garlic
$^1/_8$ teaspoon salad herb blend (optional)

Directions:
1. Combine all the ingredients in a bottle, mix and chill.
2. Remove the clove of garlic before serving.

Crohn's Disease and IBS:
Eat in moderation. Use Splenda.
Sugar 3 gms; **Fat** 7 gms

Diabetes:
Use Splenda in place of sugar in this recipe.
Carbs 13 gms; **Calories** 39

Heart Disease:
Eliminate the salt. Use the Splenda.
Sodium 1 mg; **Cholesterol** 0 mgs

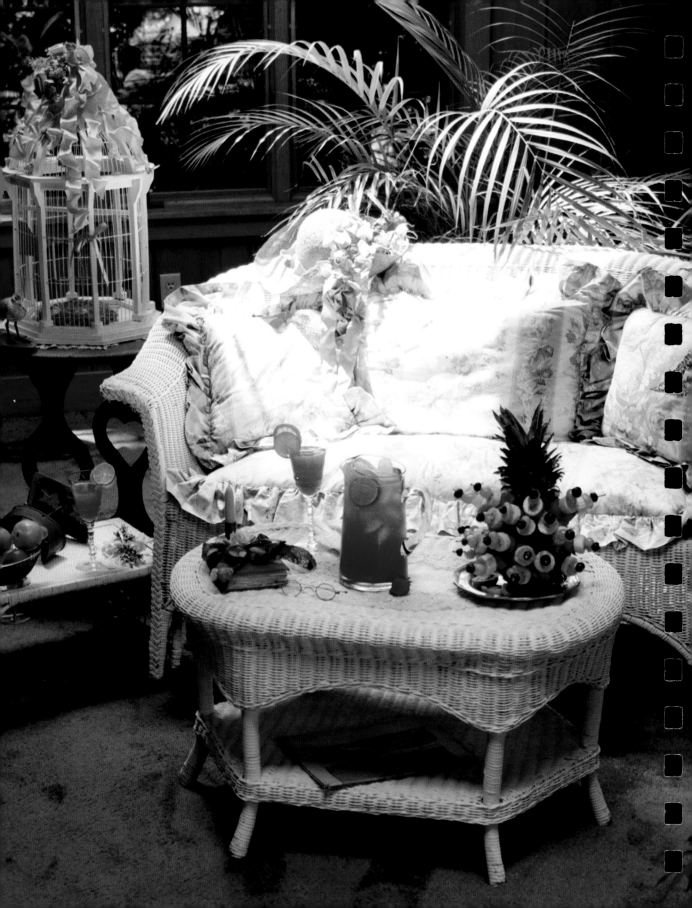

Chapter 2
FRUIT GROUP

Why eat fruits?

Fruits are probably one of the most important foods we can eat. They contain antioxidants such as beta-carotene and vitamins A and C; fruits are able to neutralize the effects of free radicals, thus slowing down the aging process. We all want to look younger, right? Fruits help us to fight infections and promote healing. They are considered a "cleansing" food and therefore should be eaten on an empty stomach or two hours after other foods have been consumed. They clean out our system by cleaning our cells, bathing our tissues and promoting the workings of our metabolic processes.

Bright colored fruits are good sources of beta-carotene. Fruits also contain their own digestive enzymes. It takes about 30 minutes for the nutrients in fruits to be released into our intestines.

Eat fresh, local fruits in season to cut down on their cost. Bananas and cantaloupe are full of potassium, calcium, phosphorous, magnesium and essential vitamins. Dried fruits are a good source of iron. By the way, did you know that canned fruits contain no preservatives? Blueberries are a wonderful source of antioxidants. I eat wild Maine blueberries every morning with a hot bowl of oatmeal. Add a glass of juice and I'm ready to meet the day.

Fruits: Buying and Storing Tips

FRESH: Bargains in season

Apples	Buy apples that are smooth, firm with unbroken surface. There should be no bruises or blemishes. Apples will keep potatoes from growing sprouts. Do you have hard brown sugar? Put a couple of slices of apple into the bag, and like magic, soft sugar.
	Storage: Place apples in a plastic bag and store in the refrigerator away from other ripening fruits. Ethylene gases in apples will over ripen other fruits. Stores for up to 3 months in the refrigerator.
Apricots	Buy apricots that have a beautiful blush, firm texture and orange yellow color.
	Storage: To ripen, store in a brown paper bag at room temperature. When ripe store for a week or two in the refrigerator.
Bananas	Bananas are ripe when yellow, taste best with brown spots, green when not ripe, brown when over ripe. I usually buy $1/2$ yellow for now and the other $1/2$ green for later. Bananas are full of potassium.
	Storage: In a fruit bowl or may be frozen for use later in banana bread, etc.

Berries   (Blackberries, blueberries and strawberries) Always shop with your nose when buying these berries. They should be bright, firm, with no mold or bruises. Locally grown will have the best flavor. The container should be free from stains. Don't wash until ready to use. Blueberries are a wonderful source of antioxidants. I pick or buy wild Maine blueberries in the summer, and freeze them for the winter months. I have Crohn's and find the small, wild Maine berries are easier for me to digest. My freezer is full of the berries.

Storage: Berries should be stored in a colander in the refrigerator, so air can circulate. Wash just before eating. Berries can be frozen. Wash and dry thoroughly, then arrange them in a single layer on a cookie sheet and freeze overnight. Place in freezer safe containers. Use frozen for baking.

Cantaloupe   Buy a cantaloupe that smells sweet. Tap on the side (like knocking on a door) 2 to 3 taps. There should be a deep thick sound. It should be orange or gold in color. The stem end should be moist with no mold. It should be firm, but not rock hard and it should feel heavy.

Storage: Store cantaloupe at room temperature until ripe, then store in the refrigerator for 2 weeks.

Cherries   Choose cherries with stems on, they will last longer. Cherries should be firm, shiny; smooth with no wrinkled skins. There are sour and sweet cherries. Cherries are usually very expensive.

Storage: If cherries are not ripe, store at room temperature. Since they dry out and absorb odors, place them in sealed plastic bags or containers. Store at room temperature or in the refrigerator crisper.

Grapefruit   Choose fruit that is smaller and thin-skinned. It should feel firm and heavy. The two varieties of grapefruit are either pink or white.

Don't take heart medication with grapefruit juice. The effects of the heart medication will be altered. Take all pills with water, unless your physician tells you otherwise.

Storage: Store grapefruits in the refrigerator or at room temperature.

Honeydew   If a honeydew is beige-skinned with green veins it is not ripe. A pale yellow color with bright lemon colored area means it is ripe. Honeydew should have a sweet smell and be firm. Do the knock test like the cantaloupe to check for ripeness.

Storage: Store at room temperature until ripe. Then store in the refrigerator.

Lemon	Lemons should have a bright yellow color. There should be no soft spots. It should have a very fresh smell. They are a good source of vitamin C. Use on salads in place of rich salad dressings. Place the used peels in the garbage disposal to eliminate odor.
	Storage: Put them in the refrigerator whole, and they will last for a couple of months.
Lime	Limes should be firm, and heavy for their size. Thin skin will yield the most juice.
	Storage: Put them in the refrigerator whole, and they will last for a couple of months.
Oranges	Oranges should be bright orange. Look for firm, heavy for its size, no blemishes or bruises, or soft spots. They are a good source of vitamin C and antioxidants.
	Storage: Store in the crisper of the refrigerator.
Peach	Buy peaches that have a sweet aroma. They should be yellow with no green. Always check for bruises and soft spots.
	Storage: Store in the refrigerator.
Pears	Purchase pears with a sweet smell and smooth, shiny skin. They should feel firm.
	Storage: Store in the refrigerator.
Plums	Plums should have a beautiful blush, firm texture, and red color.
	Storage: Store for 2-3 weeks in the refrigerator crisper.
Tangerine	A tangerine has a sweet clean fragrance. Choose bright colored skin that feels loose on the fruit. Green around the rim will not change the flavor of the tangerine.
	Storage: Store in the refrigerator.

Exotic fruits are expensive.

Guava	Guava should be tender and soft to the touch. It is the most nutritious fruit and high in vitamin C.
	Storage: Store guava at room temperature. If there is a break in the skin, store in the refrigerator.

Kiwi	A kiwi is semi-firm, but should not be too soft. The kiwi is very high in vitamin C. It is believed that kiwi helps to relieve bloating.
	Storage: Store in the refrigerator.
Papaya	A papaya is semi-firm but gives when pressed lightly. Avoid if they have too many black spots on the outside skin.
	Storage: Store in the refrigerator crisper.
Persimmons	Choose smooth, bright colored fruit that is plump.
	Storage: Store in the refrigerator.

All the fresh exotic fruits are very expensive. On a limited budget it is better to buy these fruits in cans, when on sale.

FROZEN FRUITS

Frozen fruits in the large poly bags are less expensive than the smaller packages. Divide into smaller meal size servings and freeze. Store brands and cut up pieces of fruits will cost less than whole pieces.

Frozen fruits are preserved at the peak of ripeness and freshness. If the frozen package has any discoloration or signs of being thawed, don't buy it. When you shake the frozen fruit it should separate. The frozen packages should not be soft. Melons can only be bought fresh or frozen, not canned.

Storage: Frozen fruits will keep 6-12 months in the freezer. Never re-freeze. It will cause loss of nutrients and spoilage.

CANNED FRUITS

Buy canned fruits depending on how they will be used. The price will be determined by the grade. The most expensive is Grade A, fancy. Grade B is choice and Grade C is standard. They all have the same nutritive value, but the appearance will look different. Canned fruits, like frozen fruits are harvested at proper stages of ripeness. Try to choose canned fruits in natural or light liquids.

The convenient small individual juices are hermetically sealed in containers that don't have to be refrigerated until opened. They are usually very pricey.

Never store opened cans of fruit in the refrigerator. Put them into storage containers. If buying cans or bottles of applesauce, it should be bright in color and there should be no separation of fruit and water.

Storage: Store canned fruits in a cool, dark place. They may be kept for 5 years.

STRAWBERRY-SPINACH SALAD

Ingredients: **Yields:** 6 servings
6 cups fresh spinach leaves, torn
2 cups fresh strawberries (when in season, pick your own)
1/4 cup canola oil
2 tablespoons red wine vinegar
1 tablespoon sugar or Splenda
1/2 teaspoon dried dill
1/8 teaspoon onion powder
1/8 teaspoon garlic powder
1/8 teaspoon dry mustard

Directions:
1. Place washed spinach in a bowl with the hulled, cut strawberries.
2. Combine the remaining ingredients in a screw top jar; chill.
3. Pour the chilled dressing over the mixture in the bowl.
4. Dressing may be prepared ahead of time.

If you are on blood-thinning medication, consult your physician before eating spinach. It's high in vitamin K, a blood clotting vitamin.

Crohn's Disease and IBS:
Use baby spinach leaves, they are easier to digest. Replace sugar with Splenda.
With active disease, eliminate strawberries.
Sugar 2 gms; **Fat** 4 gms

Diabetes:
Change the sugar to Splenda.
Carbs 14 gms; **Calories** 76

Heart Disease:
This is fine to eat. The spinach is high in antioxidants. Replace sugar with Splenda.
Sodium 160 mgs; **Cholesterol** 0 mgs

STRAWBERRY-BANANA JELL-O SALAD

Never use fresh or frozen kiwi, papaya or figs in Jell-O, it will not set.
I do decorate the top of the Jell-0 with kiwi, bananas and strawberries.

Ingredients: **Yields:** 6-8 servings
1 (6-ounce) package strawberry Jell-O
2 cups boiling water
1 cup orange juice
1/2 cup cold water
1 banana
1 (12-ounce) package of frozen strawberries
1 pint of low-fat sour cream or low-fat yogurt

Directions:
1. Place the Jell-O mix into a large bowl.
2. Stir 2 cups boiling water into the Jell-O.
3. Stir for 2 minutes until crystals are completely dissolved.
4. Pour in the juice and water, stir.
5. Add the frozen berries and cut up banana.
6. Pour 1/2 of mixture into a clear bowl, place in the refrigerator until it starts to gel. It will take about an hour.
7. Take mixture out of the refrigerator and cover with the yogurt.
8. Next put the other 1/2 of the Jell-O mixture on top of the yogurt.
9. Place back into the refrigerator until completely firm.
10. Decorate with bananas and kiwi.

Crohn's Disease and IBS:
Replace the juice with a low-acid orange juice. Eliminate the sour cream. Puree and strain the strawberries.
Sugar 19 gms; **Fat** 3 gms

Diabetes:
Use sugar-free Jell-O and frozen strawberries.
Carbs 14 gms; **Calories** 119

Heart Disease:
Enjoy!
Sodium 92 mgs; **Cholesterol** 0 mgs

MOM'S WALDORF SALAD

This was a favorite of ours when we were growing up in New England.

Ingredients:

Yields: 6 servings

2 cups diced unpeeled red apples
1 cup finely diced celery
½ cup coarsely cut walnuts
Mayonnaise, salad dressing, or low-fat yogurt (to suit)

Directions:

1. Mix all the above ingredients.
2. Serve on your favorite lettuce bed.

Crohn's Disease and IBS:
Peel the apples and eliminate the celery. Be sure to finely chop the nuts. Use dairy-free salad dressing.
Sugar 2 gms; **Fat** 4 gms

Diabetes:
Substitute a low-fat yogurt for the mayonnaise.
Carbs 10 gms; **Calories** 89

Heart Disease:
Use a low-fat yogurt in place of the mayonnaise. Walnuts are a good source of antioxidants.
Sodium 26 mgs; **Cholesterol** 0 mgs

MOLDED WALDORF SALAD

Pineapple is believed to settle an upset stomach.

Ingredients: **Yields:** 6 servings
1 cup boiling water
1 (11-ounce) can mandarin orange segments
1 (8¼-ounce) can pineapple chunks
1 diced medium apple
1 sliced medium banana
¼ cup coarsely chopped walnuts
Lettuce (for bed)

Directions:
1. Combine boiling water and gelatin in a medium bowl. Stir until gelatin is dissolved.
2. Mix in orange segments and its liquid, pineapple, apple, banana, and nuts.
3. Pour into a 5-cup mold.
4. Refrigerate until the Jell-O is firm.
5. Place on a bed of lettuce.

Crohn's Disease and IBS:
Peel the apple and finely chop the nuts. Eliminate the mandarin oranges.
Sugar 2 gms; **Fat** 12 gms

Diabetes:
Use sugarless Jell-O.
Carbs 16 gms; **Calories** 70

Heart Disease:
Use sugarless Jell-O.
Sodium 15 mgs; **Cholesterol** 0 mgs

BANANAS FOSTER #1 (Microwave)

Bananas are high in potassium.

Ingredients:
Yields: 6-8 servings

4 bananas
1 tablespoon lemon juice
1 tablespoon light butter or trans fat-free margarine
Pure honey to sweeten (approximately 1 tablespoon)
1/4 teaspoon cinnamon
Pinch nutmeg
2 tablespoons orange juice

Directions:
1. Peel and cut the bananas in half crosswise and then half lengthwise.
2. Brush with lemon juice and place in a microwave safe dish.
3. Combine the butter, honey, spices, and juice...drizzle over the bananas.
4. Loosely cover the bananas with white paper towels.
5. Microwave on high for 4-5 minutes.
6. Serve with vanilla frozen yogurt.

Crohn's Disease and IBS:
Use trans fat-free margarine in place of the butter, and low-acid orange juice. Serve with tofu nondairy ice cream.
Sugar 4 gms; **Fat** 1 gm

Diabetes:
Replace the honey with Splenda. Use trans fat-free margarine.
Carbs 13 gms; **Calories** 85

Heart Disease:
Use trans fat-free margarine.
Sodium 1 mgs; **Cholesterol** 0 mgs

BANANAS FOSTER #2 (In a skillet, with rum)

Ingredients: **Yields:** 4-6 servings
3 bananas
½ cup clarified butter
1 cup brown sugar or Splenda brown sugar blend
1 teaspoon pure vanilla
½ cup rum
Frozen low-fat yogurt ice cream (optional)

Directions:
1. Melt butter in skillet. Add sugar and cook over low heat, stirring constantly. Next add vanilla and cook for 3 more minutes.
2. Add bananas and continue cooking, basting bananas with sugar mixture. Add rum or rum flavoring.
3. Serve over the frozen yogurt.

Crohn's Disease and IBS:
Use tofu nondairy ice cream. Use a trans fat-free margarine.
Sugar 2 gms; **Fat** 2 gms

Diabetes:
Add molasses to the Splenda to make your own brown sugar, or buy Splenda brown sugar blend. Use a trans fat-free margarine.
Carbs 39 gms; **Calories** 99

Heart Disease:
Replace the clarified butter with a trans fat-free margarine.
Sodium 1 mg; **Cholesterol** 0 mgs

WATERMELON SWEET ONION SALSA

*Watermelon is one of the least expensive fresh fruits.
It is full of antioxidants.*

Ingredients: **Yields:** 6 servings
2 cups chopped watermelon, seeds removed
³/₄ cup chopped sweet onions
³/₄ cup canned black beans, rinsed and drained
¹/₄ cup chopped seeded jalapeno chilies
¹/₄ cup chopped cilantro or parsley
1 large clove garlic, finely chopped
1 tablespoon brown sugar
¹/₂ teaspoon salt

Directions:
1. Stir all ingredients together, cover and refrigerate.

Crohn's Disease and IBS:
Not recommended.
Sugar 1 gm; **Fat** .05 gms

Diabetes:
Make your own brown sugar using Splenda or buy Splenda brown sugar blend. Avoid too much watermelon.
Carbs 5 gms; **Calories** 29

Heart Disease:
Eliminate the salt, and use low-sodium black beans.
Sodium 3 mgs; **Cholesterol** 0 mgs

IN SEASON FRUIT SALAD

Ingredients:
½ cup strawberries
1 cup raspberries
½ cup seedless grapes
2 medium peaches
2 bananas
1 cup blueberries
1 cup cantaloupe
Lettuce leaves

Temp: Cold
Time: 5-10 minutes
Yields: 6 servings

Directions:
1. Cut up the fruit into bite size pieces, toss to mix.
2. Spoon onto lettuce leaves.
3. Serve with fresh fruit dressing. (recipe on next page)

Crohn's Disease and IBS:
Peel the peaches and eliminate the grapes. Puree and strain the strawberries and raspberries.
Sugar 11 gms; **Fat** 2 gms

Diabetes:
Enjoy and practice portion control.
Carbs 20 gms; **Calories** 91

Heart Disease:
Enjoy.
Sodium 3 mgs; **Cholesterol** 0 mgs

FRESH FRUIT DRESSING

Ingredients:
⅓ cup sugar or pure honey
¼ cup all-purpose, unbleached flour (organic)
¾ cup pineapple juice (unsweetened)
1 beaten egg or egg substitute
¼ cup lemon juice
¼ cup nonfat milk

Temp: Cold
Time: 5-10 minutes
Yields: 6 servings

Directions:
1. Combine sugar and flour in a saucepan.
2. Stir in pineapple juice.
3. Cook over medium heat, stirring constantly, about 2 minutes.
4. Cook for 2 more minutes.
5. Blend a little of the hot mixture into the egg, stirring, so the egg won't cook. (This is called tempering.) Add eggs to cooked mixture.
6. Remove from heat, add lemon juice.
7. Chill.
8. When ready to serve, beat nonfat milk and water until stiff peaks.

Crohn's Disease and IBS:
Use ⅓ cup Splenda instead of granulated sugar. Use 2 egg whites in place of whole egg.
Sugar 5 gms; **Fat** 1 gm

Diabetes:
Replace milk with skim milk and egg with 2 egg whites.
Carbs 4 gms; **Calories** 44

Heart Disease:
Use 2 egg whites in place of whole egg.
Sodium 44 mgs; **Cholesterol** 1 mg

HEALTHY FRUIT LEATHERS

Ingredients:
Apples
Apricots
Peaches
Strawberries
Raspberries
Any fruit you can blend
Any canned fruit that has been well drained

Temp: 200°
Time: Overnight (6-8 hours)
Yields: Depends on the amount of fruit you blend

Directions:
1. Peel and core fruits to be used.
2. Blend until smooth.
3. Cook for 5 minutes in a saucepan (over medium heat).
4. Place clear plastic wrap on a cookie sheet with sides.
5. Using a spoon, spread the cooked, cooled fruit as thin as possible, onto the plastic wrap. Stay away from the edges of the cookie sheet.
6. Put the cookie sheet in the oven, which is turned onto the lowest temperature (200 degrees).
7. Bake for 6-8 hours, or until fruit is dry.
8. The plastic wrap will not melt.
9. Remove from the oven and roll up in the plastic wrap.
10. Peel and eat. There is nothing but fruit, no additives.
11. The fruit leathers in the store contain many additives.

Crohn's Disease and IBS:
Enjoy. These are delicious! There is nothing but fruit in these leathers. Read the labels from store bought, they are full of sugar and coconut and palm oil. It's cheaper for the factories to add. Enjoy!

	SUGAR	FAT		SUGAR	FAT
(1) Apple	14 gms	1 gm	**1C Strawberries**	56 gms	1 gm
(1) Peach	8 gms	1 gm	**1C Raspberries**	5 gms	1 gm

Diabetes:
Enjoy, these are all natural. There is only fructose in the fruit.

	CARBS	CALORIES		CARBS	CALORIES
(1) Apple	22 gms	80	**1C Strawberries**	10 gms	44
(1) Peach	11 gms	43	**1C Raspberries**	15 gms	61

Heart Disease:
Enjoy!

	SODIUM	CHOLESTEROL		SODIUM	CHOLESTEROL
(1) Apple	0 mgs	0 mgs	**1C Strawberries**	0 mgs	0 mgs
(1) Peach	0 mgs	0 mgs	**1C Raspberries**	0 mgs	0 mgs

HEALTHY DEHYDRATED FRUIT SNACKS

My 6th grade students had so much fun making and eating these healthy snacks. Read the labels on what's in the dehydrated packages in the grocery stores. I'm sure you will agree that these are a better, healthier choice.

Ingredients:
Bananas
Apples
Pineapple
Watermelon
Strawberries

Temp: 200 degrees
Time: 6-8 hours
Yields: As many as you fix

Directions:
1. Cut banana into 1/4 inch slices.
2. Peel and core the apple and cut into 1/4 to 1/2 inch rings.
3. Pineapple, watermelon and strawberries are cut into 1/2 inch pieces.
4. Place on a nonstick cookie sheet.
5. Cook in an electric oven at 200 degrees (oven's lowest temperature). If using a gas stove, the pilot light may be enough.
6. The fruits will take about 6-9 hours to dry.
7. Store in an airtight container at room temperature.

Crohn's Disease and IBS:
These are all natural. There is only fructose in the fruit. Enjoy!

	SUGAR	FAT		SUGAR	FAT
(1) **Banana**	14 gms	1 gm	1C **Watermelon**	56 gms	1 gm
(1) **Apple**	14 gms	1 gm	1C **Strawberries**	56 gms	1 gm
1C **Pineapple**	14 gms	1 gm			

Diabetes:
Eat in moderation.

	CARBS	CALORIES		CARBS	CALORIES
(1) **Banana**	29 gms	116	1C **Watermelon**	20 gms	89
(1) **Apple**	22 gms	80	1C **Strawberries**	10 gms	44
1C **Pineapple**	19 gms	76			

Heart Disease:
Enjoy!

	SODIUM	CHOLESTEROL		SODIUM	CHOLESTEROL
(1) **Banana**	1 mg	0 mgs	1C **Pineapple**	2 mgs	0 mgs
(1) **Apple**	0 mgs	0 mgs	1C **Strawberries**	1 mg	0 mgs

FRUIT AND PASTA SALAD

Ingredients:
1 medium orange
¼ cup plain low-fat yogurt
1 teaspoon sugar or Splenda
Dash salt
¼ cup tiny bow tie pasta, cooked and drained
1 medium apple, cored and chopped
2 tablespoons sliced green onions

Time: Prep 15 minutes
Yields: 6 servings

Directions:
1. Finely shred enough orange peel to make ½ teaspoon of zest; set aside.
2. Remove the remaining peel from the orange and section orange over a bowl to catch the juice.
3. Measure 2 tablespoons of the juice.
4. In a medium mixing bowl, stir together orange peel, the 2 tablespoons of orange juice, the sugar, and the salt.
5. Mix well.
6. Add cooked pasta, chopped apples and sliced green onions; toss to coat.
7. Gently stir in orange sections.
8. Cover and chill for 2 hours.

Crohn's Disease and IBS:
Peel the apple. Use a nondairy yogurt and Splenda. Remove the onions.
Sugar 5 gms; **Fat** 1 gm

Diabetes:
Eliminate the sugar and salt. Use Splenda.
Carbs 7 gms; **Calories** 33

Heart Disease:
Eliminate the salt and use Splenda.
Sodium 6 mgs; **Cholesterol** 2 mgs

FRESH FRUIT SALAD

Ingredients:

Yields: 8-10 servings

1 cup blueberries
2 cups chunk pineapple
2 cups watermelon balls
2 cups peaches, peeled & sliced
2 cups sliced strawberries
1 cup seedless red grapes
1 fresh pear, peeled and sliced
2 bananas, peeled and sliced
2 oranges, peeled and sliced
Lemon juice
Fruit dressing

Directions:

1. Combine all fruits sprinkling lemon juice over fruit as each is prepared.
2. Chill fruits in tight container.
3. Pour fruit dressing over fruit and toss gently when ready to serve.

Fruit Dressing:

Yields: 1 cup

³/₄ cup orange juice
¹/₄ cup salad oil
1 tablespoon sugar or Splenda
¹/₂ teaspoon salt

Directions:

1. Combine ingredients.
2. Blend well and chill.
3. Serve on fruit salad.

Crohn's Disease and IBS: Not recommended.
Sugar 17 gms; **Fat** 1 gm

Diabetes: Replace sugar with Splenda. Eat sparingly.
Carbs 200 gms; **Calories** 69

Heart Disease: Eliminate the salt. Use Splenda.
Sodium 6 mgs; **Cholesterol** 2 mgs

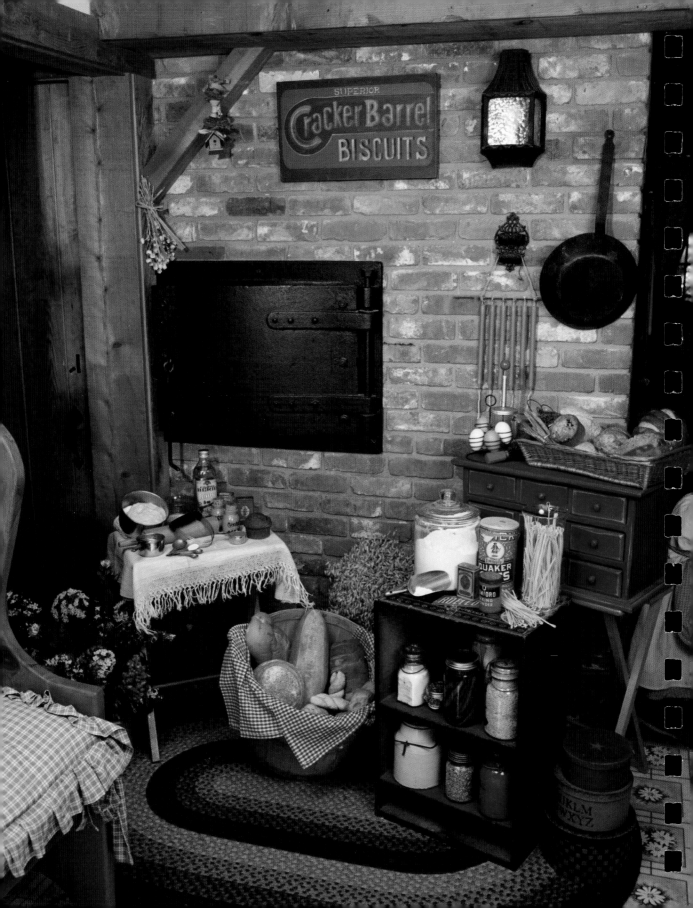

Chapter 3
BREAD, CEREAL, RICE, AND PASTA GROUP
(Whole Grained)

Why eat foods from the bread, cereal, rice, and pasta group?

Manna! The Bread of Life! Around the world, countless generations of societies, and some empires, have relied upon the ability to grow and produce grains, breads, rice, and other members of this family of foods. This staple has been subsumed into religious ceremonies which continue to this day. "Breaking bread" is an almost universal expression of greeting and comfort.

And, for good reason! Whole grained breads and cereal products provide us with necessary B complex vitamins. Thiamin, riboflavin, and niacin are essential for a healthy diet. Our ability to process the carbohydrates found in grains, breads, cereals, and rice into sugars keeps our brains and muscles functioning. The fiber in these essential foods help keep our systems flushed of toxins. Since many important nutrients are removed in the milling and refining process of grains, the Council on Food and Nutrition of the American Medical Association and many nutrition experts set up standards for restoring these lost nutrients in the foods that we eat. Whiter products indicate more refining. There are many varieties of flour. A few are bread, whole grain, cake, pastry, spelt, self-rising, bleached, and unbleached. Avoid enriched. It means the nutrients have been removed, only a few re-added.

Everyone I know enjoys the mouth-watering smells of freshly baked breads and other baked goods. And we all have those treasured memories of childhood kitchens wafting with the smells of those glorious treats. In this chapter, you will find simple, easy, delicious, and cost-effective recipes which will bring back those childhood memories, and help you make new ones for your family and friends. Easy to make, delicious to eat, and gentle on the budget, the breads, buns, pancakes, rice dishes, biscuits and pastas contained here will enhance your diet, and reawaken your senses to the gifts that this food group contains! But most of all, they are delicious. Enjoy!

BUYING

- Read labels when buying flour, rice, macaroni, cereal, bread, and other grain products. Make sure they are whole grained products.
- Don't be misled by false advertising when choosing whole grain cereals. There should be 2 grams of fiber per 100 calories. The front of the cereal box may say whole grain, but read the ingredient label to make sure that the first ingredient is whole grain.
- Buy day old bread and put it in the freezer and it will become soft again. Preferably, buy whole grain bread flour to make your own bread.

- Cereals that need to be cooked cost less than dry cereals. Oatmeal is very high in thiamin and fiber and an excellent buy. Sugar coated ready-to-eat cereals are very expensive and less nutritious. Large boxes of cooking cereals are the best buy. Examples include oatmeal, hominy grits, cream of rice, and cream of wheat cereals. Labels provide nutrient information.

- Some of the more healthy choices for grain products are bagels, pasta, noodles, corn tortillas, pita bread, corn bread, oatmeal, wheat germ and air-popped popcorn. Biscuits and muffins you bake yourself and have control of the ingredients, make a healthy choice.

- Some poorer food choices are doughnuts, pastries, croissants, taco shells, and popcorn in butter or oil.

STORAGE

Make sure all grain products are stored in dry, tightly sealed containers. This will expand the shelf life and prevent problems with infestation of weevils, or other pests. Store packages of popcorn in the freezer. I find that more corn pops when they are frozen. Did you know that brown rice has a shorter shelf life than white rice because the fat in the bran will spoil?

HINTS

When preparing baking pans for quick breads, only grease the bottom, so the batter will be able to cling to the pan. Use vegetable spray because it contains less fat.

When cooking pasta, rubbing a little oil around the top rim of the pot will prevent it from boiling over. A few drops of oil added to the water will do the same. The only problem with adding the oil directly to the pasta is that it will keep the sauce from sticking to the pasta. Did you know that fresh pasta takes only a few minutes to cook, as opposed to dried pasta?

When making yeast bread, rinse the mixing bowl with warm water and check the water temperature with the back of the hand, it should be lukewarm before adding yeast. The water temperature should be 105 to 115 degrees F. If the water is too hot it will kill the yeast; too cold and the yeast will not be activated. Do not use Splenda sweetener to activate the yeast, it won't work.

Always wash your hands before and after handling baker's yeast, as it's an active yeast culture. "Proof" the yeast to make sure it's a live culture, especially if the yeast is old. When using regular yeast, not instant, add it to the water (110 degrees) called for in the recipe. Add one tablespoon of sugar and wait for the mixture to "proof", form bubbles. If no bubbles, start over again with new yeast.

ANADAMA BREAD

Ingredients:
2 cups hot water
$\frac{1}{2}$ cup cornmeal
$\frac{1}{2}$ cup molasses
2 tablespoons shortening
2 teaspoons salt
1 package active dry yeast
$\frac{1}{4}$ cup lukewarm water
About 6 cups whole wheat flour (organic)

Temp: 325°
Time: 20 minutes
Yields: 2 loaves

Directions:
1. Bring water to boil.
2. Add cornmeal slowly.
3. Cook mixture for a few minutes.
4. Add molasses, salt and shortening.
5. Cook together until ingredients are well mixed.
6. Turn mixture into bowl. Allow to cool to lukewarm.
7. While cooling, measure $\frac{1}{4}$ cup lukewarm water, dissolve yeast in this.
8. When first mixture is lukewarm, add dissolved yeast.
9. Start adding flour.
10. When mixture makes stiff dough, turn out onto a lightly floured surface. Start kneading.
11. Add more flour as needed.
12. Place dough into greased bowl. Cover, place in warm spot until it doubles in size. Poke dough down with 2 fingers about $\frac{1}{2}$ inch into the dough. If the holes remain, the dough is ready. Let rise one more time.
13. Turn dough onto floured surface. Add more flour if necessary. Let dough rest about 10 minutes.
14. Make into two loaves and place into greased loaf pans.
15. Let rise until double in size.
16. Bake for 10 minutes at 450°. Reduce heat to 325° and bake for 20 minutes.
17. When bread has baked enough, it will sound hollow when tapped on the bottom.
18. Butter tops of loaves while still hot. It will keep the crust soft.

Crohn's Disease and IBS:
Use all-purpose, unbleached flour.
Sugar 3 gms; **Fat** 2 gms

Diabetes: Enjoy!
Carbs 6 gms; **Calories** 2

Heart Disease: Use a salt substitute.
Sodium 1 mg; **Cholesterol** 0 mgs

There is a story that goes with this bread. It seems there was a fisherman who had to cook his own food because his wife was lazy. She would only fix him cornmeal and he wanted some home made bread. He added some molasses, yeast and flour to the cornmeal and made his own bread, and said, "Anna, damn her!" The town folks decided to call the bread, "Anadama".

100% WHOLE GRAIN BREAD

Ingredients:

1 cup water

1 cup nonfat milk

2 tablespoons butter or trans fat-free margarine

$\frac{1}{4}$ cup molasses

$1\frac{1}{2}$ teaspoons salt

2 packages active dry yeast

$5\frac{1}{2}$ to $6\frac{1}{2}$ cups whole grain flour (organic)

Temp: 350°
Time: 35 minutes
Yields: 2 loaves

Directions:

1. Combine water, milk and butter or margarine in saucepan. Heat until lukewarm. (110°)
2. Pour in mixing bowl with the yeast.
3. Add honey or molasses, salt, and two cups whole grain flour.
4. Beat mixture with electric mixer for two minutes.
5. Gradually add the remainder of the flour, stirring by hand, until the dough pulls cleanly away from the sides of the bowl.
6. Place dough on floured board. Knead for 8 to 10 minutes.
7. Place in oiled bowl. Let rise for $1\frac{1}{2}$ hours in warm place.
8. Divide dough in half, shape into two loaves.
9. Place into greased loaf pans.
10. Let rise for one hour in a warm place.
11. Bake until the bread sounds hollow when tapped on the bottom.
12. When baked, brush top with butter or margarine.

Crohn's Disease and IBS:
In place of the milk, use nondairy milk. Use all-purpose, unbleached flour.
Sugar 5 gms; **Fat** 2 gms

Diabetes:
Use skim milk in place of whole milk.
Carbs 4 gms; **Calories** 17

Heart Disease:
Use only 1 teaspoon salt and heart-safe margarine. The yeast needs the salt and sugar to be activated.
Sodium 1 mg; **Cholesterol** 0 mgs

HOT CROSS BUNS

Ingredients:
4 to 5 cups of all-purpose, unbleached flour (organic)
$1/3$ cup sugar or baking Splenda
$1/2$ teaspoon salt
$1^1/4$ teaspoon cinnamon
1 package active dry yeast
1 cup low-fat milk
$1/2$ stick low-fat margarine
2 eggs, room temperature
$3/4$ cup seedless raisins
1 egg white (for top glaze)
2 tablespoons cold water

Temp: 375°
Time: 20-25 minutes
Yields: 18 buns

Directions:
1. In large mixing bowl, mix $1^1/4$ cups flour, sugar, salt, cinnamon and undissolved yeast.
2. Combine milk and margarine in saucepan. Heat over low heat until liquid is warm. (110 to 115 degrees)
3. Gradually add mixture to dry ingredients. Beat for 2 minutes. Scrape bowl occasionally.
4. Add eggs and $1/2$ cup flour. Beat at high speed for 2 minutes.
5. Stir in enough flour to make dough soft.
6. Turn onto floured surface and knead 8 to 10 minutes.
7. Place in greased bowl, turn to grease top.
8. Cover. Let rise for 1 hour.
9. Punch down. Knead in raisins.
10. Divide dough into 18 equal pieces. Form into balls.
11. Place balls in 2 well greased 8-inch round cake pans.
12. Combine egg yolk and water. Brush top of buns with mixture.
13. Cover. Let rise 1 hour.
14. Bake. Remove from the oven and let cool.
15. When just warm, frost with Confectioner's Sugar Frosting (recipe on next page).

Crohn's Disease and IBS: Eliminate the raisins, use nondairy milk, and substitute 4 egg whites in place of 2 whole eggs.
Sugar 2 gms; **Fat** 3 gms

Diabetes: You will need 2 teaspoons of granulated sugar to activate the yeast. Use low-fat milk.
Carbs 5 gms; **Calories** 40

Heart Disease: In place of the whole eggs, substitute 4 egg whites. Use only heart-safe margarine. There will be a red heart on the label.
Sodium 7 mgs; **Cholesterol** 0 mgs

CONFECTIONER'S SUGAR FROSTING

These buns are a tradition at Easter.

Ingredients:
1¼ cup confectioner's sugar
⅛ cup trans fat-free margarine
¼ teaspoon pure vanilla extract
1 tablespoon low-fat milk or skim milk

Directions:
1. Mix all the ingredients in a small mixing bowl.
2. Drizzle over the hot cross buns in a cross design.

Crohn's Disease and IBS:
Replace the milk with a nondairy milk.
Sugar 2 gm; **Fat** 3 gms

Diabetes:
Splenda should work well in this recipe. Use skim milk.
Carbs 3 gms; **Calories** 2

Heart Disease:
Use the Splenda in this recipe. Use skim milk.
Sodium 1 mg; **Cholesterol** 0 mgs

ECOLOGY BREAD

Yeast is a living plant and makes the bread rise. High heat will kill the yeast. Water should be between 105°F and 115°F.

Ingredients:
1 cup water
1 cup low-fat milk
1/4 cup canola oil
1 cup rolled oats
2 teaspoons salt
1/2 cup molasses
1 package active dry yeast
4 1/2 to 5 1/2 cups whole wheat flour (organic)

Temp: 350°
Time: 35 minutes
Yields: 2 loaves

Directions:
1. Combine water and milk in saucepan and bring to boil. Add oil.
2. Shut off heat; add oats and stir.
3. Cool mixture to lukewarm. Never add yeast to hot liquid.
4. Add yeast, salt, and molasses to cooled mixture.
5. Beat with a spoon for two minutes.
6. Add flour, a little at a time.
7. Divide dough in half.
8. Knead dough on lightly floured board. (It will take about 8 to 10 minutes.) If necessary, sprinkle the board with more flour.
9. Place dough into greased bowls.
10. Cover; let dough rise in warm place until it doubles in size, about 1 hour.
11. Form into loaves.
12. Place in loaf pans and bake.
13. Remove loaves and lay on a cooling rack on its side.

Crohn's Disease and IBS:
Exchange the milk to nondairy milk. Use all-purpose, unbleached flour.
Sugar 3 gms; **Fat** 2 gms

Diabetes:
Enjoy!
Carbs 6 gms; **Calories** 50

Heart Disease:
Use only 1 teaspoon salt.
Sodium 3 mgs; **Cholesterol** 0 mgs

ONE BOWL LOW-CHOLESTEROL BREAD

Let rise in a warm place free from any draft.

Ingredients:
7 to 8 cups unsifted whole wheat flour (organic)
2 tablespoons sugar or baking Splenda
2 teaspoons salt
1 package active dry yeast
1 tablespoon softened, low-fat margarine or butter
2½ cups very warm water

Temp: 400°
Time: 40-45 minutes
Yields: 2 loaves

Directions:
1. In large mixing bowl, thoroughly mix 2½ cups flour, sugar, salt, and dissolved yeast.
2. Add butter or margarine.
3. Gradually add warm water to dry ingredients and beat 2 minutes at medium speed. Scrape bowl occasionally.
4. Add ¾ cup flour, enough to make thick batter.
5. Beat at high speed 2 minutes. Scrape bowl occasionally.
6. Stir in enough additional flour to make a soft dough.
7. Turn onto a lightly floured board; knead until smooth and elastic, about 8 to 10 minutes.
8. Place in greased bowl; turn to grease top.
9. Cover and let rise in warm place until doubled in size.
10. Punch down dough; turn onto lightly floured board.
11. Divide in half, shape into two loaves.
12. Place in two greased loaf pans.
13. Let rise 1 hour, bake.

Crohn's Disease and IBS:
Use all-purpose, unbleached flour.
Sugar 2 gms; **Fat** 3 gms

Diabetes:
Use only 1 tablespoon sugar and 1 tablespoon of Splenda. You need at least 2 teaspoons of granulated sugar to activate the yeast.
Carbs 2 gms; **Calories** 20

Heart Disease:
Use a heart-safe margarine. There will be a heart shaped logo on the package. The salt, along with the sugar, is needed to activate the yeast.
Sodium 120 mgs; **Cholesterol** 0 mgs

ICE BOX BUTTER BUNS

A college friend, Sandy, gave this recipe to me.
It was passed down from generation to generation in Sandy's family.

Ingredients:
1 package active dry yeast
2 tablespoons warm water (110 degrees)
½ cup sugar or baking Splenda
1 egg beaten
2 cups warm low-fat milk
1 teaspoon salt
½ cup melted trans fat-free margarine
6 cups all-purpose, unbleached flour (organic)

Temp: 400°–425°
Time: 12–15 minutes
Yields: 48 small rolls

Directions:
1. Dissolve yeast in warm water. (Rinse bowl with warm water. Water needs to stay warm to properly dissolve yeast.)
2. Add sugar and beaten egg.
3. Mix in salt, milk, and margarine.
4. Gradually mix in flour. MIX, DO NOT KNEAD!
5. Let mixture stand uncovered in refrigerator for 8 hours.
6. Shape into desired rolls.
7. Bake.

Crohn's Disease and IBS:
Use nondairy milk. Replace the whole egg with egg substitute or 2 egg whites. Use baking Splenda.
Sugar 2 gms; **Fat** 3 gms

Diabetes:
Replace the whole egg with egg substitute or 4 egg whites.
Carbs 2 gms; **Calories** 24

Heart Disease:
Replace the whole egg with egg substitute or 2 egg whites.
Sodium 17 mgs; **Cholesterol** 0 mgs

QUICK BREADS (Are quick to make)

There are 3 types of quick breads:

1. Pour Batter: waffles, crepes, pancakes, and popovers (these contain equal amounts of flour to liquid)

2. Drop batter: muffins and loaf breads (twice the flour to liquid)

3. Soft dough: cinnamon rolls, biscuits (3 times the flour to liquid)

All of these batters contain basically the same ingredients: flour, milk, leavening agent (baking soda, baking powder, cream of tartar), shortening, salt, sugar, flavoring, and eggs. The major difference is the amount of liquid to dry ingredients.

It is very important to never over mix quick breads. When you mix liquid with flour, it forms gluten. If you over develop the gluten, the batter will be too elastic. Your quick breads will be tough and muffins will have holes from the carbon dioxide. Remember, DO NOT OVER MIX!!

If a recipe says sifted flour and you don't sift, you will have 2 extra tablespoons of flour for each cup. Don't pack the cup with the flour, gently spoon it into the cup. Using a wire strainer will also work as a sifter. Sifting puts air in the flour and it takes less to fill the cup.

It's also very important to use the correct measuring cups. A glass cup is used to measure liquids. There is extra room in the cup so you don't spill the liquid. The graduated nesting cups are used for dry ingredients. Gently spoon the dry ingredients into the cup and don't shake it down. Level it off at the top with a knife.

Always allow 10 minutes to preheat an oven to reach the desired temperature.

Place a pan in the center of the oven when baking to insure even baking. There should be 2 inches on all sides of the pan for the heat to circulate evenly.

BAKING POWDER BISCUITS

Biscuits are quick and easy and require only a few ingredients. They can be used for breakfast, on top of a casserole for lunch, or part of a dessert (such as strawberry shortcake).

Ingredients:
2 cups all-purpose, unbleached flour (organic)
1 tablespoon baking powder (aluminum-free)
$^1/_2$ teaspoon salt
$^1/_3$ cup butter flavored shortening
$^3/_4$ cups low-fat milk

Temp: 450°
Time: 10 minutes
Yields: 10-12 biscuits

Directions:
1. Sift flour and then measure 2 cups.
2. Place the flour back into the sifter with the baking powder and salt.
3. Add shortening. Cut it into the flour mixture using a pastry blender or 2 knives.
4. Stir in most of the milk using a fork until the dough follows the fork around the bowl.
5. On a lightly floured surface, knead dough 10-12 times.
6. Using a rolling pin, roll out dough until it is about $^1/_2$ inch thick.
7. Cut biscuits with a floured 2$^1/_2$ inch biscuit cutter.
8. Place biscuits on an UNGREASED cookie sheet.
9. Bake. For soft sides, place biscuits close together.

Crohn's Disease and IBS:
Use nondairy milk (example: soy). Use baking Splenda.
Sugar 2 gms; **Fat** 5 gms

Diabetes:
Substitute sugar with Splenda. Use low-fat or skim milk.
Carbs 8 gms; **Calories** 70

Heart Disease:
Use baking Splenda and skim milk.
Sodium 0 mgs; **Cholesterol** 9 mgs

85

SKY HIGH BISCUITS

These biscuits are great for desserts and shortcakes.

Ingredients:
2 cups all-purpose, unbleached flour (organic)
1 cup whole wheat flour
4½ teaspoons baking powder (aluminum-free)
1 tablespoon sugar or Splenda
¾ teaspoon cream of tartar
¾ cup trans fat-free margarine
1 egg or 2 egg whites
1 cup low-fat milk

Temp: 450°
Time: 12-15 minutes
Yields: 20 biscuits

Directions:
1. Combine flour, baking powder, sugar and cream of tartar in bowl.
2. Cut in margarine with pastry blender or 2 knives until it looks like corn meal.
3. Add egg and milk. Stir only until dry ingredients become wet.
4. Knead lightly on floured surface.
5. Roll out dough to 1-inch thickness.
6. Place on lightly greased cookie sheet.
7. Bake.

Crohn's Disease and IBS:
Substitute low-fat milk with nondairy milk. Replace whole egg with 2 egg whites.
Replace sugar with Splenda.
Sugar 1 gm; **Fat** 1 gm

Diabetes:
Use Splenda in place of granulated sugar. Replace the whole egg with 2 egg whites.
Carbs 30 gms; **Calories** 44

Heart Disease:
Use 2 egg whites in place of the whole egg.
Sodium 9 mgs; **Cholesterol** 0 mgs

CINNAMON ROLLS

Ingredients:
2 cups sifted all-purpose, unbleached flour (organic)
1 tablespoon baking powder (aluminum-free)
¼ teaspoon salt
⅓ cup butter flavored shortening
¾ cup low-fat milk

Filling:
3 tablespoons soft, Smart Balance margarine
¼ cup sugar or Splenda
2 teaspoons of cinnamon

Temp: 400°
Time: 10-12 minutes
Yields: 12 rolls

Directions:
1. Sift and then measure 2 cups flour. Place the sifted flour back into the sifter with the baking powder and salt. It will be well blended when sifted together.
2. Using a pastry blender or 2 knives, cut in the shortening so it looks like corn meal.
3. Using a fork, stir in a little milk at a time, mixture should form a ball. Caution, you may not need all of the milk.
4. Place the dough on a lightly floured surface and knead the dough.
5. KNEAD the dough by pressing, folding, and turning 6-10 times.
6. With a lightly floured rolling pin, roll the dough ¼ inch thick in a rectangular shape.
7. Spread the margarine over the top of the dough with the back of a spoon.
8. Mix sugar and cinnamon together and sprinkle over the margarine.
9. Beginning at the long edge, roll the dough tightly. Seal by pinching the edges together.
10. Cut into approximately ½ inch slices (with a knife or dental floss). There should be 12 equal pieces. Place into greased muffin pan, cut side down.
11. Bake.

Crohn's Disease and IBS:
Use nondairy milk. Use Splenda in place of sugar.
Sugar 2 gms; **Fat** 3 gms

Diabetes:
Use Splenda in place of sugar.
Carbs 8 gms; **Calories** 77

Heart Disease:
Use Splenda in place of sugar.
Sodium 4 mgs; **Cholesterol** 0 mgs

LOW-FAT BRAN MUFFINS

*This recipe is well tested. My husband Andy
makes these muffins twice a week.*

Ingredients:
1 cup whole wheat flour (organic)
½ teaspoon baking powder (aluminum-free)
½ teaspoon baking soda
½ teaspoon cinnamon
1½ cups 100% all-bran cereal
1¼ cups low-fat milk
⅓ cup packed brown sugar or Splenda brown sugar blend
1 egg or 2 egg whites
½ cup applesauce* (sugar-free)
½ cup raisins, optional

The applesauce in this recipe takes the place of oil.

Temp: 400°
Time: 18 minutes
Yields: 12 muffins

Directions:
1. Preheat oven.
2. Mix flour, baking powder, baking soda, and cinnamon in mixing bowl.
3. In second bowl, mix bran cereal, milk, and sugar.
4. Let cereal mixture set in bowl for at least 5 minutes.
5. Add egg and applesauce to cereal mixture.
6. Add wet mixture to dry ingredients. Mix until blended.
7. Do not over mix batter. Mixture should be lumpy.
8. Spray muffin pan with nonstick spray. Fill ⅔ full with mixture.
9. Bake.
10. Eat warm.

Crohn's Disease and IBS:
When making this recipe use a nondairy milk. Use Splenda brown sugar blend.
Use all-purpose, unbleached flour.
Sugar 5 gms; **Fat** 3 gms

Diabetes:
Use Splenda brown sugar blend. Always use skim milk.
Carbs 11 gms; **Calories** 51

Heart Disease:
Replace the whole egg with 2 egg whites. Always use skim milk. Use Splenda brown
sugar blend.
Sodium 79 mgs; **Cholesterol** 0 mgs

HEALTHY ORANGE BRAN FLAX MUFFINS

Ingredients:
1½ cups oat bran
1 cup whole wheat flour (organic)
1 cup flaxseed, ground
1 cup wheat bran
1 tablespoon baking powder (aluminum-free)
½ teaspoon salt
2 oranges, quartered and seeded
1 cup brown sugar or Splenda brown sugar blend
1 cup buttermilk
½ cup canola oil
2 eggs or 4 egg whites
1 teaspoon baking soda
1½ cups golden raisins

Temp: 375°
Time: 18-20 minutes
Yields: 24 muffins

Directions:
1. Preheat oven.
2. Coat two 12-cup muffin pans with cooking spray.
3. In a large bowl, combine oat bran, flour, flaxseed, wheat bran, baking powder, and salt. Set aside.
4. In a blender, combine oranges, brown sugar, buttermilk, oil, eggs, and baking soda. Blend well.
5. Pour orange juice mixture into dry ingredients. Mix until well blended.
6. Stir in raisins.
7. Divide batter evenly among muffin cups.
8. Bake.
9. Cool in pan for 5 minutes. Place on a cooking rack.

Crohn's Disease and IBS:
Not recommended.
Sugar 6 gms; **Fat** 3 gms

Diabetes:
Use skim milk and 4 egg whites.
Carbs 11 gms; **Calories** 38

Heart Disease:
Eliminate salt. Replace buttermilk with skim milk. Use the 4 egg whites.
Sodium 8 mgs; **Cholesterol** 0 mgs

ECONOMICAL CORN BREAD

Ingredients:

1 cup sifted, all-purpose, unbleached flour (organic)

¼ cup nonfat dry milk

3 tablespoons sugar or baking Splenda

3½ teaspoons baking powder (aluminum-free)

1 teaspoon salt

1 cup cornmeal (Quaker whole grain Arrowhead Mills)

1 egg or 2 egg whites

1 cup water

¼ cup canola oil

Temp: 425°
Time: 25 minutes
Yields: 20 squares

Directions:

1. Mix flour, dry milk, sugar, baking powder, and salt.
2. Add cornmeal and mix well.
3. Combine water and liquid shortening, add to dry mixture.
4. Add egg.
5. Do not over mix.
6. Pour into well greased 8x8x2 baking pan.
7. Bake.

Crohn's Disease and IBS:
The recipe is ok to eat when symptom-free. Replace sugar with baking Splenda. Use egg whites and a nondairy milk.
Sugar 3 gms; **Fat** 3 gms

Diabetes:
Substitute sugar with Splenda.
Carbs 8 gms; **Calories** 35

Heart Disease:
Replace the whole egg with 2 egg whites. Use ½ teaspoon of salt.
Sodium 12 mgs; **Cholesterol** 0 mgs

CORN BREAD

This recipe came from a second grade teacher celebrating Thanksgiving with her students. The children were dressed up as Pilgrims and Indians and shared a meal that our forefathers would have eaten together as a sign of peace.

Ingredients:
1/2 cup all-purpose, unbleached flour (organic)
1/2 cup cornmeal (Quaker Arrowhead Mills Brand)
2 teaspoons baking powder (aluminum-free)
1/2 teaspoon salt
2 tablespoons sugar or baking Splenda
1 egg, slightly beaten or 2 egg whites
1/2 cup low-fat milk
1 1/2 tablespoons light butter or low-fat margarine
1 (8 1/2-ounce) can cream-style corn, blended

Temp: 425°
Time: 25-30 minutes
Yields: 8 servings

Directions:
1. Sift all dry ingredients. Place into mixing bowl.
2. Add beaten egg and milk to dry ingredients.
3. Add margarine and blended corn to mixture.
4. Stir mixture only slightly.
5. Place in greased 8x8x2 baking pan.
6. Bake.

Crohn's Disease and IBS:
Not recommended.
Sugar 2 gms; **Fat** 2 gms

Diabetes:
Sugar can be replaced with Splenda. Corn is high in sugar. Use Smart Balance light margarine. Always use skim milk.
Carbs 14 gms; **Calories** 85

Heart Disease:
Use 2 egg whites in place of the whole egg. Replace heart-safe margarine for the butter. Use baking powder and a low-sodium corn. Always use skim milk.
Sodium 32 mgs; **Cholesterol** 0 mgs

BANANA BREAD

Ingredients:
2½ cups all-purpose, unbleached flour (organic)
½ cup brown sugar or Splenda brown sugar blend
½ cup granulated sugar or baking Splenda
3½ teaspoons baking powder (aluminum-free)
3 tablespoons salad oil
1 teaspoon pure vanilla extract
⅓ cup low-fat milk
1 egg or 2 egg whites
3 medium ripe bananas*

Temp: 350°
Time: 60 minutes
Yields: 1 loaf

Directions:
1. Grease bottom of 9x5x3 loaf pan.
2. Mash bananas in mixing bowl.
3. Add sugars, oil, vanilla, and milk to bananas. Add eggs.
4. Mix in baking powder and a little flour at a time to liquid ingredients.
5. Pour into loaf pan and bake.

Use bananas that are dark in color for the most flavor. Bananas also freeze well.

Crohn's Disease and IBS:
Replace milk with nondairy milk. Use baking Splenda and Splenda brown sugar blend.
Use 2 egg whites in place of the whole egg.
Sugar 7 gms; **Fat** 2 gms

Diabetes:
Substitute the granulated sugar with baking Splenda and Splenda brown sugar blend.
Replace the whole egg with 2 egg whites.
Carbs 6 gms; **Calories** 550 loaf or 36 per slice

Heart Disease:
Replace the whole egg with 2 egg whites. Use baking Splenda and Splenda brown sugar blend.
Sodium 7 mgs; **Cholesterol** 0 mgs

DUMPLINGS

Ingredients:
1½ cups sifted, all-purpose, unbleached flour (organic)
2 teaspoons baking powder (aluminum-free)
¾ teaspoon salt
3 tablespoons shortening
¾ cup 1% milk

Temp: Medium heat
Time: 20 minutes
Yields: 12 servings

Directions:
1. Sift together the flour, baking powder, and salt.
2. Cut in the shortening with a pastry blender.
3. Stir in ¾ cup of milk until blended.
4. Drop spoonfuls onto chicken or beef in boiling stock.
5. Cook slowly, uncovered, for 10 minutes and covered another 10 minutes.
6. Remove hot meat and dumplings to a warmed platter.
7. Cover with chicken or beef gravy.

Shortening can't be replaced with liquid oils unless the recipe says so.

Crohn's Disease and IBS:
Use nondairy milk in place of milk.
Sugar 1 gm; **Fat** 10 gms

Diabetes:
Substitute 1% milk with skim milk.
Carbs 1 gm; **Calories** 10

Heart Disease:
Use only ½ teaspoon of salt. Substitute 1% milk with skim milk.
Sodium 2 mgs; **Cholesterol** 0 mgs

GERMAN OVEN PANCAKES

Ingredients:
½ cup all-purpose, unbleached flour (organic)
½ teaspoon nutmeg
3 eggs or egg substitute
¾ cup 1% low-fat milk
2 tablespoons vegetable oil spread

Temp: 425°
Time: 10 minutes, then change to 325° for 10 minutes
Yields: 2 pie plates full

Directions:
1. Combine above ingredients and mix with rotary beater or blender.
2. Place into 2 well greased pie plates.
3. Bake. DO NOT PEEK! Pancake will deflate.
4. Serve with maple syrup or fresh fruit.

Crohn's Disease and IBS:
Replace milk with nondairy milk. Use egg substitute.
Sugar 1 gm; **Fat** 2 gms

Diabetes:
Use skim milk.
Carbs 5 gms; **Calories** 14

Heart Disease:
Replace whole eggs with egg substitute. The egg substitute carton will tell you how many eggs are in the package.
Sodium 15 mgs; **Cholesterol** 0 mgs

CREPES

Ingredients:
1 cup low-fat milk
$^2/_3$ cup all-purpose, unbleached flour (organic)
1 egg or 2 egg whites
1 tablespoon canola oil
$^1/_8$ teaspoon salt
$^1/_2$ teaspoon pure vanilla extract

Temp: Medium heat
Time: Until brown
Yields: 12 servings

Dessert crepes:
Omit the salt and add 2 tablespoons sugar or Splenda, plus $^1/_2$ teaspoon vanilla.

Directions:
1. Combine egg, milk, flour, oil, vanilla, and salt in a bowl.
2. Beat with wire whisk until well mixed.
3. Heat a lightly buttered 6-inch nonstick pan.
4. Tilt pan to spread butter.
5. Remove from heat. Pour 2 tablespoons batter into pan.
6. Return to heat. Brown on one side only.
7. Make the remainder of crepes until batter is gone.

After cooking, the crepes may be frozen. Wrap by putting waxed paper between them. Place in freezer bags to be used at a later date. To serve, leave at room temperature for one hour to thaw. Fill with one tablespoon of fruit or favorite filling. Roll each into cylinders.

Crohn's Disease and IBS:
Replace low-fat milk with nondairy milk.
Sugar 1 gm; **Fat** 2 gms

Diabetes:
Use the 2 egg whites in place of the whole egg. Replace sugar with Splenda. Use skim milk in place of low-fat milk.
Carbs 4 gms; **Calories** 17

Heart Disease:
Use the 2 egg whites in place of the whole egg. Eliminate the salt. Use skim milk in place of low-fat milk.
Sodium 28 mgs; **Cholesterol** 0 mgs

APPLE PUFFED PANCAKES

Ingredients:

3 eggs or egg substitute

¾ cup low-fat milk

½ cup all-purpose, unbleached flour (organic)

1½ tablespoons granulated sugar or baking Splenda

½ teaspoon pure vanilla extract

¼ teaspoon cinnamon

¼ cup trans fat-free margarine

1 large apple peeled and thinly sliced

Enough Splenda brown sugar blend to sprinkle on the top of the pancake

Temp: 425°
Time: 20 minutes
Yields: 4 servings

Directions:

1. Preheat oven for 10 minutes.
2. Place eggs, milk, flour, granulated sugar, vanilla, and cinnamon into a blender.
3. Melt the margarine in an 11x7¼ baking dish in the oven.
4. Add the apple slices to the margarine and place back into the oven until the margarine starts to sizzle...don't let it brown.
5. Take the baking dish out of the oven and pour batter over the apples.
6. Sprinkle with brown sugar.
7. Bake in the middle of the oven for 20 minutes.
8. Serve with strawberry sauce.

Strawberry Sauce:

Heat a package of frozen strawberries with 1 tablespoon of orange juice until it is warm. Serve over the pancake.

Crohn's Disease and IBS:

Replace milk with a nondairy milk. Use egg substitute. Replace sugar with baking Splenda.
Sugar 13 gms; **Fat** 4 gms

Diabetes:

Replace the sugar with Splenda.
Carbs 11 gms; **Calories** 107

Heart Disease:

Substitute margarine with heart-safe margarine. Use an egg substitute.
Sodium 92 mgs; **Cholesterol** 0 mgs

QUICK BROWN BREAD

Ingredients:
2 cups whole grain flour (organic)
1 teaspoon salt
$\frac{1}{2}$ teaspoon baking soda
$1\frac{1}{2}$ teaspoon baking powder (aluminum-free)
1 egg or 2 egg whites
1 cup reduced-fat sour cream
$\frac{1}{2}$ cup molasses
$\frac{1}{2}$ cup canola oil

Temp: 350°
Time: 30 minutes
Yields: 1 loaf

Directions:
1. Mix flour, salt, baking soda, and baking powder thoroughly in mixing bowl.
2. Beat egg. Add sour milk, molasses, shortening and mix.
3. Add liquid mixture to dry ingredients.
4. Stir just enough to mix ingredients.
5. Pour into greased bread pan.
6. Bake.
7. Serve with baked beans.

Crohn's Disease and IBS:
Replace sour milk with nondairy milk, and eliminate baked beans. Use 2 egg whites in place of whole eggs. Use all-purpose, unbleached flour.
Sugar 1 gm; **Fat** 2 gms

Diabetes:
Enjoy!
Carbs 3 gms; **Calories** 45

Heart Disease:
Use $\frac{1}{2}$ teaspoon of salt, or eliminate altogether. Use 2 egg whites in place of whole eggs.
Sodium 6.5 mgs; **Cholesterol** 0 mgs

POPOVERS

Ingredients:
1¼ cups 1% milk
1¼ cups all-purpose,
  unbleached flour (organic)
½ teaspoon salt
3 eggs or egg substitute

Temp: 425°
Time: 20 minutes, then decrease temp
    to 325° for additional 15-20 minutes
Yields: 6 servings

Directions:
1. Preheat oven.
2. With wire whisk beat milk, flour, and salt. Do not over mix.
3. Beat in eggs one at a time until well blended.
4. Pour into popover cups. Fill about ¾ full. Use nonstick steel popover pans that do not have to be greased. (Grease well if not using nonstick steel popover pans.)
5. Bake...do not peek!

Crohn's Disease and IBS:
Replace the milk with nondairy milk. Use egg substitute.
Sugar 2.5 gms; **Fat** 1 gm

Diabetes:
Use egg substitute and skim milk.
Carbs 2 gms; **Calories** 31

Heart Disease:
Eliminate the salt and use egg substitute in place of the whole eggs. Use skim milk.
Sodium 45 mgs; **Cholesterol** 2 mgs

FRENCH TOAST

Ingredients:
8 slices of whole grain or Italian bread
3 large eggs or egg substitute
$^3/_4$ cup low-fat milk
1 teaspoon pure vanilla extract
1 teaspoon cinnamon
Pinch of nutmeg (optional)

Temp: Medium heat
Time: 10 minutes
Yield: 4-5 servings

Directions:
1. Spread out the bread slices in a glass baking dish.
2. In a medium bowl, mix eggs, milk, vanilla, cinnamon, and nutmeg.
3. Pour over bread slices and let it sit until you are ready.
4. Heat your griddle, melt a small amount of butter spray and add the soaked bread.
5. Cook until brown on one side, turn and cook about 2 minutes.
6. Transfer to plates and cover with your favorite syrup or fruit.

Crohn's Disease and IBS:
Use vanilla tofu or soy dairy milk. Use egg substitute. Select Italian bread.
Sugar 4 gms; **Fat** 1.5 gms

Diabetes:
Use gluten-free bread and skim milk.
Carbs 8 gms; **Calories** 78

Heart Disease:
Replace the eggs with egg substitute or egg whites. Use skim milk and no sodium bread.
Sodium 70 mgs; **Cholesterol** 0 mgs

BASIC WAFFLES

Ingredients:
2 cups all-purpose, unbleached flour (organic)
3 tablespoons sugar or baking Splenda
1 tablespoon baking powder (aluminum-free)
1 teaspoon salt
2 eggs or 4 egg whites
¼ cup melted butter or trans fat-free margarine
2 cups low-fat milk, as needed

Temp: Turn on waffle iron
Time: 5 minutes
Yields: 8-9 waffles

Directions:
1. Place the flour, sugar, baking powder, and salt in a small bowl. Stir with a wire whisk to evenly distribute the ingredients. Add the melted butter, eggs, and about 1½ cups of milk. Blend with a wire whisk until smooth and free from lumps. Batter should be thick but still pour slowly from a ladle or measuring cup. Add more milk as needed to obtain a thick but pourable consistency. If the batter becomes too thin, stir in a teaspoon or two of additional flour.
2. Preheat the waffle iron to "ready" temperature.
3. Pour a generous ⅓ cup of batter onto the preheated waffle griddle. Close the lid; press it down tightly to level batter. Bake until the signal indicates the waffle is done.
4. Remove the waffle and place on a wire rack for about 30 seconds then serve.*

Note: Waffles may be kept warm in a preheated 300° oven for 5 to 10 minutes but their consistency may change. Batter can be held overnight under refrigeration. If it thickens, add milk to restore to the desired consistency.

Crohn's Disease and IBS:
Replace milk with nondairy milk. (I use soy.)
Sugar 4 gms; **Fat** 15 gms

Diabetes:
Use Splenda and low-fat skim milk.
Carbs 17 gms; **Calories** 66

Heart Disease:
Eliminate salt. Use egg substitute to replace the whole eggs. Use Splenda and low-fat skim milk.
Sodium 54 mgs; **Cholesterol** 0 mgs

HOMEMADE GRANOLA

Ingredients:
4 cups quick cooking rolled oats
1 cup sunflower nuts
$1/2$ cup slivered almonds
$1/2$ cup unsalted raw pumpkin seeds
$1/2$ cup wheat germ
$1/4$ cup extra virgin olive oil
$1/4$ cup honey
$1/3$ cup water
1 cup finely chopped, dried apricots
1 cup finely chopped prunes
1 cup raisins

Temp: 250°
Time: 30 minutes
Yields: 10 cups

Directions:
1. Pre-heat oven.
2. Lightly grease 2 cookie sheets.
3. Combine oats, sunflower nuts, almonds, pumpkin seeds, and wheat germ into medium bowl.
4. Mix the oil and honey in a small bowl. Add to above mixture.
5. Stir until well mixed.
6. Sprinkle the water, a tablespoon at a time over the mixture as it is tossed.
7. Equally divide the mixture onto the 2 cookie sheets.
8. Bake for 1 hour. Stir every 15 minutes.
9. Next, stir in the apricots, prunes and raisins. Put pan back into the oven for 15 additional minutes.
10. Fruit will be slightly soft, not dry.
11. Cool and store in a tightly covered container.

Crohn's Disease and IBS:
Not recommended.
Sugar 2 gms; **Fat** 13 gms

Diabetes:
Eliminate the wheat germ.
Carbs 54 gms; **Calories** 372

Heart Disease:
Good to eat. This is a very healthy recipe for most people.
Sodium 5 mgs; **Cholesterol** 0 mgs

HOMEMADE SEASONED BREAD CRUMBS

Ingredients:
1 pound Italian or whole wheat bread
1 teaspoon crushed dried thyme
1 teaspoon crushed dried oregano
1 teaspoon crushed dried basil
1/4 teaspoon pepper

Temp: 300°
Time: 15 minutes
Yields: 1 1/2 cups

Directions:
1. Cut Italian bread in half lengthwise.
2. Cut each half into slices, then cut slices into 1/2" cubes.
3. Place cubes in a shallow baking dish.
4. Bake until cubes are golden brown (15 minutes) stirring several times.
5. Remove from oven and cool completely.
6. Mix cubes with the crushed spices.
7. Blend in a food processor or blender, until fine.
8. Store in a tightly sealed container.
9. May be stored in the refrigerator or freezer.

Crohn's Disease and IBS:
Use Italian bread.
Sugar 2 gms; **Fat** 2 gms

Diabetes:
Enjoy. Use low-carb bread.
Carbs 20 gms; **Calories** 105

Heart Disease:
Use low-sodium bread.
Sodium 110 mgs; **Cholesterol** 0 mgs

APPLE BREAD STUFFING

Ingredients:
3/4 cup chopped onions
3/4 cup finely diced celery
1 minced clove of garlic
Cooking spray
7 cups toasted bread cubes (whole grain)
3 cups finely chopped and peeled Macintosh apples
2 eggs or egg substitute
3/4 cup skim milk
1/2 cup butter or trans fat-free margarine
Pepper to taste
2 tablespoons poultry seasoning (or to taste)
2 tablespoons chopped parsley

Temp: 350°
Time: 30 minutes
Yields: 8-9 cups

Directions:
1. In a 10-inch skillet, sauté the onions and celery in cooking spray until tender.
2. Place cooked mixture in a large bowl and cool.
3. Add the bread cubes and chopped apples.
4. Whip eggs and add to mixture.
5. Scald milk and margarine.
6. Cool and add the milk and margarine to the bowl.
7. Mix in the pepper, poultry seasoning, and parsley.
8. To prevent possible bacterial contamination, it is advised that the stuffing be cooked separately in a greased casserole dish.
9. If stuffing is cooked in the chicken or turkey, place cold stuffing into the bird, cook immediately. Remove stuffing when completely cooked.

Crohn's Disease and IBS:
Use a nondairy milk, trans fat-free margarine, and egg substitute.
Sugar 5 gms; **Fat** 2 gms

Diabetes:
Choose trans fat-free margarine and low-carb bread.
Carbs 14 gms; **Calories** 43

Heart Disease:
Use egg substitute. Use Promise margarine.
Sodium 22 mgs; **Cholesterol** 0 mgs

WHY EAT RICE?

Rice is the food source for two-thirds of our planet's population. This grain is highly nutritious, versatile, low cost, and easy to prepare. It is considered one of the highest quality proteins and contains all of the eight essential amino acids. As a complex carbohydrate, rice helps to fuel the body. It's stored up in the muscles and released as energy when needed.

Rice is wonderful for people with special diets. It contains no cholesterol, fat, or sodium and is non-allergenic and gluten-free.

BUYING

There are a variety of different kinds of rice. One of the healthiest is brown rice. Brown rice is an unmilled rice that has the hull removed, but retains the bran layer. This allows the grain to retain more of the vitamins, minerals, and fiber. The bran is the barrier to heat and moisture. It takes about 45 minutes to cook. Brown rice is higher in fat and carbohydrates than white rice, however, the nutritional benefits outweigh this fact.

Some of the common rice used is long, medium, and short grains. Long grain rice cooks up light and fluffy. One cup of rice is used with $1^3/_4$ cup water. Rice will triple in size when cooked.

STORAGE

Rice is a convenient food and is easy to store. Once opened, rice should be stored in an airtight container. Brown rice, if kept for more than a month, should be stored in the refrigerator or freezer due to the oil contained in the bran layer. Cooked rice is stored in an airtight container for a week in the refrigerator or in the freezer for six months.

NUTRITIOUS BROWN RICE (Baked in the Oven)

Baking brown rice in the oven is considered the best way for having perfect rice. Always make sure you use the exact measurements.

Ingredients:
6 cups water
1 cup brown rice
2 teaspoons extra virgin olive oil
1 teaspoon salt

Temp: 375°
Time: 80 minutes
Yields: 4 servings

Brown rice baked in the oven:
1. Preheat the oven to 375°F.
2. Place the rack in the middle of the oven.
3. Spread the rice in an 8-inch square glass baking dish.
4. In a covered saucepan, on top of the stove, boil water and olive oil.
5. Pour the boiling water over the rice in the baking pan.
6. Sprinkle rice with the salt.
7. Tightly cover the baking dish with foil.
8. Cook for one hour, or until tender.
9. Remove the foil and stir rice with a fork.
10. Cover rice dish with a clean cloth, and let rice stand for 5 minutes.
11. Uncover the rice for another 5 minutes, and serve.

Crohn's Disease and IBS: Fine to eat.
Sugar 0 gms; **Fat** 1 gm

Diabetes: Fine to eat.
Carbs 11 gms; **Calories** 67

Heart Disease: Eliminate the salt.
Sodium 1 mg; **Cholesterol** 0 mgs

NUTRITIOUS BROWN RICE (Stove Top)

Ingredients:
6 cups water
1 cup brown rice
2 teaspoons extra virgin olive oil
1 teaspoon salt

Temp: Boil and simmer
Time: 30 minutes
Yields: 4 servings

Top of stove brown rice:
1. Boil water in large pan.
2. Stir in rice, salt, and oil.
3. Simmer uncovered for about 30 minutes.
4. Drain rice and place in top of double boiler. Fill bottom of broiler with 1½ inches of water.
5. Place top portion with rice onto bottom of broiler.
6. Cover and steam rice until tender, usually 6 to 10 minutes.
7. Place cooked rice in a warm serving bowl.

Crohn's Disease and IBS: Fine to eat.
Sugar 1 gm; **Fat** 1 gm

Diabetes: Fine to eat.
Carbs 11 gms; **Calories** 67

Heart Disease: Eliminate the salt.
Sodium 1 mg; **Cholesterol** 0 mgs

PERFECT WHITE RICE

Ingredients:
2 teaspoons extra virgin olive oil
1 cup long grain unconverted white rice
1½ cups water
½ teaspoon salt

Temp: Medium heat, 2 minutes
Time: Low heat, 15 minutes
Yields: 3 cups

Directions:
1. In saucepan heat olive oil.
2. Add rice and stir for 2 minutes.
3. Add water and salt. Bring mixture to a boil.
4. Turn temperature to low and cover, continue to cook for 15 minutes.
5. Turn heat off. Leave covered on stove for 15 minutes.

Crohn's Disease and IBS:
This is part of the BRAT diet, (bananas, rice, applesauce, and toast), and good for people with Crohn's disease. It helps if you are having a rough day and living in the bathroom.
Sugar 1 gm; **Fat** 6 gms

Diabetes:
Rice is fine for diabetics.
Carbs 15 mgs; **Calories** 86

Heart Disease:
Eliminate the salt.
Sodium 0 mgs; **Cholesterol** 0 mgs

RICE PILAF

Ingredients:
1½ cups fresh mushrooms
6 green onions
3 tablespoons butter or trans fat-free margarine
2⅛ cups water
1 cup regular long grain rice
¾ medium bell pepper
¾ teaspoon salt
¾ teaspoon dried sage, crushed
2 tablespoons parsley, snipped

Temp: Microwave
Time: 14-16 minutes
Yields: 6 servings

Directions:
1. Combine mushrooms, onions, and butter or margarine in a ½ quart casserole dish.
2. Microwave uncovered on 100% power for 1½ to 2½ minutes or until vegetables are tender.
3. Stir in water, rice, bell pepper strips, salt, and sage.
4. Microwave covered on 100% power for 12 to 14 minutes or until rice is tender and liquid is absorbed, stirring once.
5. Stir in parsley.
6. Let stand covered for 5 minutes.

Crohn's Disease and IBS:
Peel the green pepper. Use a trans fat-free margarine.
Sugar 0 gms; **Fat** 2 gms

Diabetes:
Fine to eat. Use a trans fat-free margarine.
Carbs 17 gms; **Calories** 109

Heart Disease:
Eliminate the salt. Use Promise margarine.
Sodium 46 mgs; **Cholesterol** 0 mgs

BASIC FRESH PASTA DOUGH

If you rub some oil along the top inside rim of the pot, the pasta won't boil over. Fresh pasta cooks more quickly than packaged pasta.

Ingredients:
1½ cups all-purpose, unbleached flour (organic)
1½ cups semolina or durum flour
1½ teaspoons salt
1½ tablespoons extra virgin olive oil
4 beaten eggs or egg substitute

Temp: Boiling (212°)
Time: 3-4 minutes
Yield: 6 plus servings

Directions:
1. Place all ingredients except eggs into food processor.
2. Add eggs a bit at a time while pulsing.
3. When dough forms into pellets enough egg has been added.
4. Turn dough onto work surface and knead together into stiff mass.
5. Cover and let rest for 15 minutes before rolling and cutting into desired shape.
6. Cut dough into 4 equal pieces.
7. Work with 1 piece at a time, while keeping remaining dough covered.
8. Roll dough out on a floured surface as thin as possible, or use a pasta machine at thinnest setting.
9. Drape cut strips over dowel rods suspended between two chairs to slightly dry (approximately 5 minutes).
10. Fill a large pot with 4 quarts of water, per pound of pasta.
11. Oil along the top rim of pot so water won't boil over.
12. Bring the water to a rolling boil and add the pasta.
13. Stir occasionally to prevent the pasta from sticking.
14. Drain and serve with your favorite sauce.

Crohn's Disease and IBS:
Use egg substitute. Enjoy!
Sugar 3 gms; **Fat** 2 gms

Diabetes:
Use egg substitute.
Carbs 40 gms; **Calories** 127

Heart Disease:
Eliminate the salt and use egg substitute in place of the whole eggs.
Sodium 23 mgs; **Cholesterol** 0 mgs

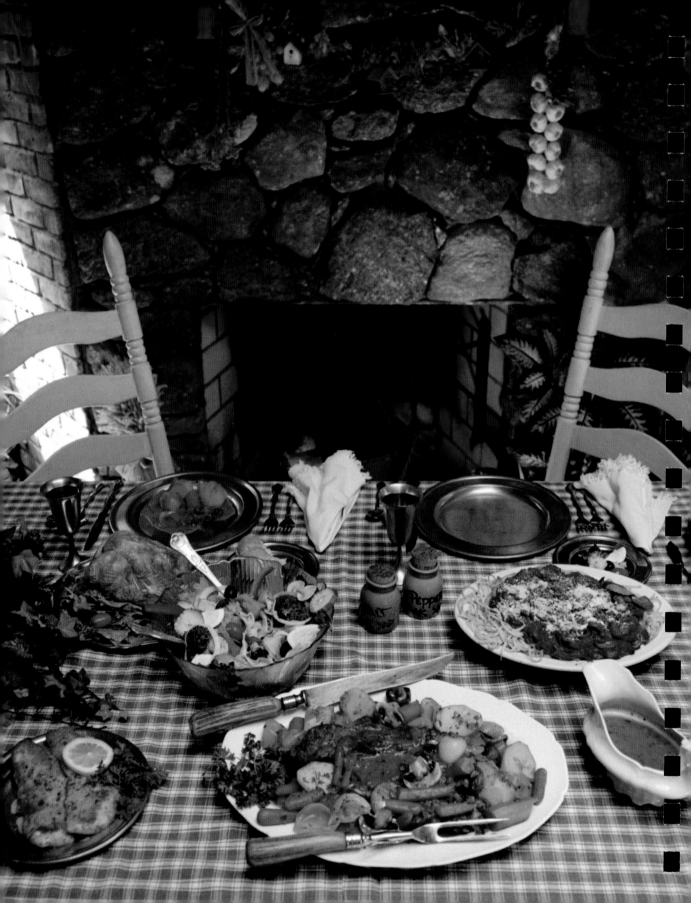

Chapter 4
MEAT GROUP

Why eat foods from the meat group?

Meats supply us with our greatest source of protein, essential for building and maintaining body tissues. Without them we would have a lowered resistance to infection, mental and physical fatigue.

The following beef/veal, pork, and lamb charts show the basic retail cuts from each of the wholesale cuts. All the retail low-cost cuts are colored blue and your high-cost cuts are colored red. The names of the retail cuts may vary in different parts of the country, but the wholesale cuts are usually the same. The location of the cut will greatly determine the cost. For example, the forequarter of the beef is where you would find the low-cost cuts of beef. If chuck is on the meat label you know the price should be low.

Any animal part that moves a great deal (around the shoulder and legs) has more connective tissue and is tougher. It is usually lower in cost and requires slow moist heat cooking in order to break down the connective tissue. Pounding, grinding, scoring, and cubing also help to tenderize meat. The low-cost cuts have the same food value as the more expensive cut. The major difference is that the expensive cuts are more tender. With proper cooking, low-cost cuts can be just as tender and tasty as high-cost cuts.

In order to know what to buy when you reach the market, it is a must to learn how to recognize the different cuts.

Beef, lamb, and veal all have the same muscle and bone structure. The difference is the color of the meats and size of the cuts.

Since meat is perishable, it should be stored properly in the refrigerator or freezer. Remove from store packaging and rewrap securely or store in an airtight container. To prevent freezer burn use freezer-safe wrap. Always defrost in the refrigerator, not on the counter top.

COOKING TECHNIQUES
Meat (Beef/Veal, Pork, and Lamb)

The two classifications of meat cookery: 1. Dry Heat Cooking
                                              2. Moist Heat Cooking

DRY HEAT COOKING

A. Roasting
Roast meat at a low temperature and always use a meat thermometer. There is less shrinkage and loss of protein, thiamine, and vitamin B. The only loss is some water and fat. The following steps will insure a tender, nutritious roast.

1. Place meat on a rack with the fat side up.
2. Gently sprinkle the fat with salt and pepper. Salt brings out the juices in meat, so only salt the fat.
3. Insert a meat thermometer into the center of the roast away from the bone and fat.
4. Roast uncovered in a 325°-350° oven.
5. DO NOT ADD WATER OR SEAR MEAT!

Remove from oven when done. Let meat juices set before carving – about 10 minutes. This allows juices to be absorbed back into the meat.

B. Broiling
1. Place meat on broiler rack about 2″ from the heat.
2. Cut through outside fat 1″ apart to keep edges from curling.
3. Set oven regulator to broil.
4. Leave door slightly ajar for electric stove and closed for a gas stove.
5. Broil until meat is brown then turn it over and brown the other side.
   Rare – about 5 minutes each side for a 1″ steak
   Med – about 6 minutes each side
   Well done – about 8 minutes each side
6. Season and serve on a hot plate.

C. Frying
1. Add cooking spray to a skillet.
2. Use medium heat on top of range.
3. DO NOT ADD WATER AND DO NOT COVER.
4. Turn meat occasionally and cook it slowly. Meat should be dried.
5. Pan fry when meat has very little fat or is breaded or floured.

MOIST HEAT COOKING (for low-cost cuts of meat)

This method of cooking is used for less expensive and tougher cuts of meat. The liquid helps to break down the connective tissue that causes meat to be tough.

A. Braising or Pot Roasting

1. Cover meat with seasoned flour (salt, pepper, and flour).
2. Brown meat in a little cooking spray.
3. Add a little liquid; if it boils away add more.
4. Cover pan tightly and cook over low heat for 2-3 hours if pot-roasting, and 1-2 hours if braising.
5. Vegetables may be added the last ½ hour.

B. Stewing

1. Have beef, lamb cut into 1 or 2-inch cubes.
2. Roll meat in seasoned flour.
3. Brown on all sides in hot cooking spray.
4. Partially cover meat with water.
5. Cover pan and cook slowly until meat is tender, simmer but do not boil.
6. Add cut-up vegetables the last ½ hour.
7. Thicken gravy with Wondra or flour and water.

WHOLESALE BEEF/VEAL CUTS

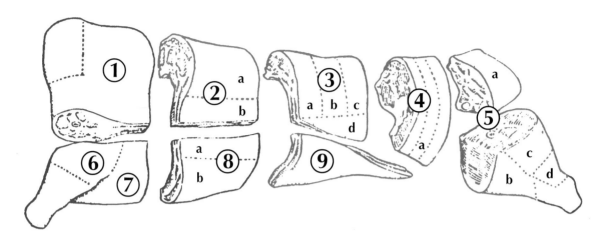

LOW-COST RETAIL CUTS: COLORED BLUE; HIGH-COST RETAIL CUTS: COLORED RED

1. CHUCK
a. Stew Beef
b. Hamburger
c. Chuck Roast and Steak
d. Yankee Pot Roast (boneless)

2. RIB
a. Rib Roast
b. Short Rib

3. SHORT LOIN
a. Club Steak
b. T-bone Steak
c. Porterhouse Steak (is a better buy than a T-bone because it has a bigger tenderloin)
d. Filet Mignon cuts are located in this area

4. LOIN
a. Sirloin

5. RUMP (round)
a. Rump Roast
b. Sirloin Tip Roast
c. Round Roast and Steak
d. Eye of Round

6. FORE SHANK
a. Shank

7. BRISKET
a. Corned Beef

8. SHORT PLATE
a. Stew Beef
b. Hamburger

9. FLANK
a. Steak

By products...miscellaneous:
- Bones
- Tripe - Stomach
- Beef Liver
- Beef Heart
- Oxtail

Veal is a young calf and is very expensive.

HINTS

With modern technology, meat is packed so it arrives to local markets just about every day.

Your retail meat cuts contain the same food value. The only difference is that your higher cost cuts are more tender. With proper preparation your low cost cuts can be just as tender. A serving of meat is the size of a deck of cards or the palm of your hand.

Ground turkey contains less fat than ground chicken or beef.

Make sure you have a cutting board that is used just for meat. It can be cleaned with 1 teaspoon of bleach in hot water.

HOW TO STRETCH GROUND BEEF OR TURKEY

To 1 pound of lean ground beef or turkey add any of the following:
2 slices of moistened bread
or
$1/2$ cup oatmeal
or
$1/4$ cup crushed dry cereal

SIMMERED BEEF SHANKS

Ingredients:
2 tablespoons all-purpose, unbleached flour (organic)
1 tablespoon salt
1/4 teaspoon pepper
3-4 pounds crosscut beef shanks
1 tablespoon canola oil
1 cup low-sodium tomato juice
1/2 teaspoon dried basil, crushed (optional)
4 medium potatoes, pared and quartered
2 tablespoons Wondra (quick mixing flour for sauces and gravy)

Temp: Medium heat
Time: 30-40 minutes
Yields: 6 servings

Directions:
1. Combine 2 tablespoons flour, salt, and pepper in a paper bag. Add beef shanks and shake.
2. Brown meat in hot canola oil.
3. Add tomato juice and basil.
4. Cover and simmer for 1 1/2 hours.
5. Add potatoes, cover and simmer 30-40 minutes, until potatoes are tender.
6. Remove meat and potatoes, skim off excess fat from juice.
7. Add enough water to juice to make 1 cup of liquid.
8. Mix together 1/2 cup cold water and 2 tablespoons Wondra (quick mixing flour), stir into juices.
9. Cook and stir until thick and bubbly.
10. Serve with potatoes.

Crohn's Disease and IBS:
Use extra virgin olive oil. Enjoy.
Sugar 3 gms; **Fat** 14 gms

Diabetes:
Substitute flour with rice or soy flour. Use extra virgin olive oil.
Carbs 30 gms; **Calories** 122

Heart Disease:
Eliminate the salt, and use extra virgin olive oil.
Sodium 15 mgs; **Cholesterol** 11 mgs

CHUCK STEAK CASSEROLE

Ingredients:
1½ pounds chuck steak
2 teaspoons salt
Dash pepper
1 teaspoon paprika
2 tablespoons all-purpose, unbleached flour (organic)
2 tablespoons canola or extra virgin olive oil
1 medium onion, sliced
4 small potatoes, sliced
1 cup canned crushed tomatoes
1 tablespoon ketchup (organic)

Temp: 350°
Time: 1¼ hours
Yields: 6-8 servings

Directions:
1. Cut steak into 4 pieces.
2. Season with salt, paprika, pepper, and coat with flour.
3. Brown in hot oil in heavy skillet.
4. Place browned meat into a casserole dish.
5. Put onions and sliced potatoes over the top.
6. Mix tomatoes and ketchup and pour over potatoes.
7. Cover and bake.

Crohn's Disease and IBS:
Blend the tomatoes before using.
Sugar 1.8 gms; **Fat** 5.5 gms

Diabetes:
Use tomato paste in place of ketchup. Ketchup contains sugar.
Carbs 18 gms; **Calories** 76

Heart Disease:
Use tomato paste in place of ketchup. Use basil or thyme in place of salt.
Sodium 10 mgs; **Cholesterol** 11 mgs

BASIC LEFTOVER MIXTURE (Ground Beef or Turkey)

Yields: 2 one pound packages
of leftover beef mixture

Ingredients:

1 pound lean ground beef or turkey (93%, plus 2 tablespoons canola oil)
2 cups bread crumbs from Italian bread (soaked in water and drained)
1 teaspoon salt
¼ teaspoon pepper
3 tablespoons low-fat cream of mushroom soup or leftover gravy

Directions:

1. Combine the above ingredients.
2. Make up 2 packages of leftover mixture and freeze them.

NOTE: The following two recipes can be made from this Basic Leftover Mixture.

CABBAGE ROLL-UPS

Ingredients:
12 cabbage leaves
1 package leftover beef mixture (see recipe on page 118)
1 chopped medium onion
$\frac{1}{2}$ clove garlic minced
$\frac{1}{4}$ cup chopped button mushrooms
1 (15-ounce) can crushed tomatoes
$\frac{1}{2}$ cup cooked instant brown rice
Salt and pepper to taste
$\frac{1}{4}$ cup grated low-fat Parmesan cheese

Temp: 350°
Time: 45 minutes
Yields: 6 servings

Directions:
1. Place cabbage leaves in boiling water. Cover and leave for about 10 minutes. Leaves should be limp. Remove and dry leaves.
2. In a saucepan brown the meat mixture, chopped onions, garlic, and mushrooms.
3. Add $\frac{1}{2}$ can of crushed tomatoes into the mixture and stir.
4. Mix in the cooked rice.
5. Place equal amounts of meat mixture at stem end of each leaf. Roll leaf around beef mixture and tuck under the roll.
6. Place the cabbage rolls in an 8x8x2 ungreased square pan.
7. Pour the remaining crushed tomatoes over the cabbage rolls.
8. Cover and bake.
9. Sprinkle with the Parmesan cheese.

Crohn's Disease and IBS:
Not recommended.
Sugar 5 gms; **Fat** 7 gms

Diabetes:
Use a low-carbohydrate unseasoned breadcrumb made from Italian bread.
Carbs 6 gms; **Calories** 100

Heart Disease:
Eliminate the salt. Use a low-sodium cream of mushroom soup.
Sodium 71 mgs; **Cholesterol** 6 mgs

MEAT TURNOVERS

Ingredients:
1 package leftover beef mixture (see recipe on page 118)

Temp: 350°
Time: 20 minutes
Yields: 4 servings

One Crust Oil Pastry:
2 cups all-purpose, unbleached flour (organic)
2 to 3 pinches baking powder (aluminum-free)
$^2/_3$ cup canola oil
Pinch of salt
$^1/_3$ cup cold orange juice

Directions:
1. Mix flour, oil, salt, and baking powder until particles are the size of a small pea.
2. Add orange juice a tablespoon at a time until the pastry forms a ball.
3. If pastry seems dry try adding a little more oil, not orange juice.
4. Gather dough into a ball.
5. Roll dough thin (about $^1/_8$" thick) and cut into four 4" squares.
6. Place equal amounts of leftover beef mixture (1 package) onto one side of the four rolled out dough squares. (Leave room to seal edges.)
7. Wet edges and seal with a fork.
8. Brush tops of turnovers with a whipped up egg for a professional look.
9. Bake.

Crohn's Disease and IBS:
Use low-acid orange juice in place of regular juice.
Sugar 1 gm; **Fat** 13 gms

Diabetes:
Eliminate the salt.
Carbs 8 gms; **Calories** 80

Heart Disease:
Eliminate the salt and enjoy!
Sodium 245 mgs; **Cholesterol** 7 mgs

AMERICAN CHOP SUEY

Ingredients:
4 cups boiling water
1⅓ cups uncooked pasta (whole grain, better choice)
½ pound lean ground beef or ground turkey
1⅓ cups canned crushed tomatoes
¼ cup low-sodium tomato sauce
¼ cup tomato paste
1 small onion
1 clove garlic, crushed
¼ cup of chopped green pepper
1 tablespoon canola or extra virgin olive oil
1 teaspoon salt
½ teaspoon pepper
Season to taste with sweet basil and Parmesan cheese

Temp: Medium heat
Time: ½ hour
Yields: 6 servings

Directions:
1. Heat water in a covered saucepan until it boils.
2. Add pasta with a pinch of salt.
3. Boil gently until pasta is tender, stir with a wooden spoon.
4. Drain thoroughly, rinse with water, and drain again.
5. While pasta is cooking, peel and chop onion, green pepper, and garlic.
6. Cook until tender, in oil.
7. Add ground meat to the onions, pepper, and garlic.
8. While cooking, keep stirring until meat is cooked.
9. Add the crushed tomatoes and tomato sauce to the meat mixture.
10. Mix in the pasta, salt, pepper, and spices.
11. Cook thoroughly on low to medium heat.

Crohn's Disease and IBS:
Finely chop the onion and green pepper. Blend the tomatoes.
Sugar 3 gms; **Fat** 5 gms

Diabetes:
Replace the pasta with brown rice pasta. Its wheat-, gluten-, and fat-free.
Carbs 20 gms; **Calories** 93

Heart Disease:
Use the brown rice pasta, it's also low in sodium. Eliminate the salt.
Sodium 28 mgs; **Cholesterol** 5 mgs

HEALTHY MEAT LOAF

Ingredients:
³/₄ pound lean ground turkey
³/₄ pound lean ground beef (93%, plus 2 tablespoons canola oil)
1 large onion, finely chopped
1 stalk celery, finely chopped
1 clove garlic, minced
¹/₂ cup bread crumbs (recipe on page 102)
2 tablespoons Mrs. Dash (salt-free seasoning blend)
2 tablespoons tomato paste
¹/₂ teaspoon pepper
2 egg whites
1 tablespoon skim milk
1 cup tomato puree

Temp: 375°
Time: 1 hour
Yields: 6 servings

Directions:
1. Heat oven to 375°.
2. Grease an 8¹/₂x4¹/₂x2¹/₂ loaf pan. (Or use cooking spray. It contains less fat.)
3. Sauté onions, celery, and garlic until soft, not brown. Cool (easier to digest).
4. Mix all the ingredients together until well blended.
5. Spread in the loaf pan with a rubber scraper.
6. Bake uncovered.
7. Cover with tomato sauce the last 10 minutes.

TO COOK MEAT LOAF MORE QUICKLY

Cook in muffin tins for 15 minutes at 375°
or three 5³/₄ x 3 x 2¹/₈ loaf pans for 30 minutes at 375°.

Crohn's Disease and IBS: Use nondairy milk in place of skim milk.
Sugar 4 gms; **Fat** 1 gm

Diabetes: Use rice based crumbs.
Carbs 10 gms; **Calories** 52

Heart Disease: Eliminate the salt.
Sodium 70 mgs; **Cholesterol** 0 mgs

YANKEE POT ROAST

Ingredients:
All-purpose, unbleached flour (organic)
4 pound pot roast
1 small turnip, cut up
6 carrots
6 small boiling onions
6 potatoes
1 tablespoon parsley
Any leftover vegetables (peas, string beans, etc.)
2 tablespoons all-purpose, unbleached flour (organic)
¼ cup water
Salt and pepper to taste

Temp: Medium
Time: 3 hours (on top of stove)
Yields: 8+ servings

Directions:
1. Dredge a 4 pound pot roast in flour. Cook in heavy, greased skillet.
2. When brown, add approximately 3 cups boiling water, cover and simmer 3 hours. Add vegetables, last hour.
3. Mix 2 tablespoons flour in ¼ cup water to make gravy. Add to pot roast, stirring constantly. May top with biscuits or dumplings in place of flour and water mixture.

Crohn's Disease and IBS:
Eliminate the turnip, it's too hard to digest.
Sugar 4 gms; **Fat** 7 gms

Diabetes:
Substitute rice flour in place of flour.
Carbs 28 gms; **Calories** 150

Heart Disease:
Eliminate the salt.
Sodium 17 mgs; **Cholesterol** 44 mgs

CHILI

Ingredients:
¾ cup chopped onion
2 cloves crushed garlic
1 pound lean ground beef (93%) or ground turkey
1 tablespoon canola oil (to add moisture to lean beef, do not use with turkey)
Cooking spray
½ cup chopped celery
1 (16-ounce) can whole tomatoes
1 (15-ounce) can kidney or red beans drained
1 teaspoon salt
1 carrot for sweetness (remove when chili is cooked)
1 tablespoon chili powder (add more if you like it hot)
1 teaspoon low-sodium Worcestershire sauce
Cooking spray

Temp: Medium to medium high heat
Time: 1 hour, 15 minutes
Yields: 5-6 servings

Directions:
1. In a non-stick 2-quart saucepan, add cooking spray. Brown the onion, garlic, and meat. Drain excessive liquid.
2. Next, stir in the tomatoes, celery, chili powder, salt, carrot, and Worcestershire sauce.
3. Cover and simmer for 1 hour.
4. Stir in the beans and bring to a boil.
5. Simmer for 15 minutes, stir occasionally.

Crohn's Disease and IBS:
Not recommended.
Sugar 1 gm; **Fat** 9 gms

Diabetes:
Eliminate the salt. Enjoy.
Carbs 8.6 gms; **Calories** 37

Heart Disease:
Use ground turkey in place of beef. Eliminate the salt.
Sodium 199 mgs; **Cholesterol** 5 mgs

ORIGINAL SWEDISH MEATBALLS

Ingredients:
¼ cup skim milk
1 cup whole grain bread cubes (save leftover toast)
1½ pounds 93% lean ground beef or ground turkey
3 tablespoons canola oil (use only with beef)
¼ cup finely chopped onions
½ cup mashed potatoes (leftover from the potato skins recipe – see page 51)
2 egg whites
Cooking spray

Temp: Medium heat
Time: 35 minutes
Yields: 6 servings

And a mixture of:
1 teaspoon salt
½ teaspoon pepper
½ teaspoon brown sugar or Splenda brown sugar blend
¼ teaspoon allspice
2 tablespoons all-purpose, unbleached flour (organic)
½ cup beef broth, canned or homemade (see page 209)
2 teaspoons tomato paste
¼ cup light butter or trans fat-free margarine
1 cup low-fat sour cream or yogurt

Directions:
1. Combine milk and bread cubes. Let stand for 5 minutes, then using fingers, squeeze out excessive milk from the bread cubes.
2. Spray skillet with cooking spray and cook onions over low heat.
3. In large mixing bowl mix together meat, bread, onions, salt, pepper, brown sugar, allspice, and mashed potato.
4. Beat the eggs and add to the meat mixture.
5. Shape the meat into small meatballs.
6. In a large skillet, melt ¼ cup butter or margarine over medium heat.
7. Brown the meatballs for 5 minutes on each side.
8. Remove meatballs after browned.
9. Reduce heat and stir flour in the pan drippings.
10. Add beef broth and tomato paste, cook over medium heat until thick.
11. Add meatballs to skillet; simmer covered for 15 minutes.
12. Stir in the sour cream and serve.

Crohn's Disease and IBS: Use nondairy milk. Replace sugar with Splenda brown sugar blend. Use a trans fat-free margarine and Italian bread.
Sugar 5.8 gms; **Fat** 20 gms

Diabetes: Exchange the bread cubes with gluten-free bread. Use Splenda brown sugar blend, and a trans fat-free margarine.
Carbs 6 gms; **Calories** 382

Heart Disease: Eliminate salt. Substitute ground turkey for the beef. Use a heart-safe margarine and Splenda brown sugar blend.
Sodium 94 mgs; **Cholesterol** 33 mgs

SHEPHERD'S PIE

Ingredients:
1 pound lean ground beef (93%, plus 2 tablespoons canola oil)
1 small chopped onion
Cooking spray
1 (15¼-ounce) can cream-style corn
Mashed potatoes (5 potatoes)
Salt and pepper to taste
¼ cup low-fat milk

Temp: 325°
Time: 20 minutes
Yields: 6 servings

Directions:
1. Sauté onions and ground beef in small amount of cooking spray.
2. Place in the bottom of an 11x8x2 casserole dish.
3. Pour cream style corn over the cooked ground beef.
4. Top with mashed potatoes.
5. Bake.

Crohn's Disease and IBS:
Eliminate the corn and use a vegetable you can eat. I use cooked carrots. The low-fat milk should be replaced with nondairy milk. I use soy.
Sugar 3.6 gms; **Fat** 10 gms

Diabetes:
Replace low-fat milk with skim milk. Use no salt corn. Corn contains sugar.
Carbs 5 gms; **Calories** 75

Heart Disease:
Eliminate the salt. Use no salt corn.
Sodium 87 mgs; **Cholesterol** 20 mgs

ECONOMY LASAGNA CASSEROLE

Ingredients:
1 small chopped onion
Cooking spray or oil
1/2 teaspoon salt
1/2 teaspoon pepper
1 pound ground turkey or lean ground beef (93%, plus 2 tablespoons canola oil)
1 (1-pound, 13-ounce) can crushed tomatoes
1 (8-ounce) can tomato sauce
1/2 pound lasagna noodles (whole grain)
1/2 pound low-fat mozzarella cheese (buy whole and slice, less expensive)
1/2 pound drained low-fat, low-sodium cottage cheese (in place of ricotta cheese)
1/4 cup low-fat Parmesan cheese

Temp: 350°
Time: 20 minutes
Yields: 6-8 servings

Directions:
1. Cook onions until soft in small amount of cooking oil.
2. Brown ground meat.
3. Stir in tomatoes, tomato sauce, and seasoning. Simmer 20 minutes.
4. Cook lasagna noodles in salt water until tender, drain.
5. Pour 1/3 of sauce in 12x8x2 baking dish.
6. Cover with strips of lasagna noodles.
7. Put strips of mozzarella over lasagna noodles.
8. Place spoonfuls of cottage cheese on top.
9. Repeat layers ending with meat sauce.
10. Top with Parmesan cheese.
11. Bake.

Crohn's Disease and IBS:
Use all nondairy cheeses.
Sugar 2.5 gms; **Fat** 7.8 gms

Diabetes:
Use rice or soy lasagna noodles.
Carbs 21 gms; **Calories** 212

Heart Disease:
Select the ground turkey, rather than the beef. Eliminate the salt and use low-fat dairy products. Read the label in all low-fat products, and make sure they haven't added extra sugar to replace the fat.
Sodium 116 mgs; **Cholesterol** 20 mgs

MEAT-ZA-PIE

When using 93% ground beef instead of ground turkey, always add 2 tablespoons canola oil to moisturize. The canola oil is better for you than animal fat.

Ingredients:
½ teaspoon salt and pepper
½ cup dried whole grain breadcrumbs
⅔ cup of 1% low-fat milk
1 pound ground turkey or lean ground beef (93%, plus 2 tablespoons canola oil)
½ cup tomato sauce or paste
2 or 3 slices American cheese (cut in strips)
¼ to ½ teaspoon oregano
2 tablespoons grated Parmesan cheese

Temp: 400°
Time: 20 minutes
Yields: 5-6 servings

Directions:
1. Place beef or turkey, salt, and bread crumbs in a 9" pie plate.
2. Add milk and mix together.
3. Spread mixture evenly over the bottom of the plate, raising the rim about ½" high on the sides of the plate.
4. Spread the tomato paste mixture over the meat mixture.
5. Arrange the cheese strips in criss-cross pattern over the top.
6. Sprinkle with Parmesan and oregano over the top.
7. Bake.

Crohn's Disease and IBS:
Use nondairy milk. Replace the American cheese with a soy cheese.
Sugar 7.3 gms; **Fat** 9 gms

Diabetes:
Use soy or rice breadcrumbs. Replace the cheese with a low-fat brand.
Carbs 22 gms; **Calories** 100

Heart Disease:
Eliminate the salt, use low-fat cheese, and only use turkey.
Sodium 100 mgs; **Cholesterol** 27 mgs

BEEF MARINADE

Great for stew meat used as shish kabobs (see recipe on page 130).

Ingredients:
½ cup salad oil
¼ cup vinegar
¼ cup chopped onions
1 teaspoon salt
Dash of pepper
2 teaspoon low-sodium Worcestershire sauce

Temp: Medium heat
Time: 10 minutes
Yields: 1 cup

Directions:
1. Combine all ingredients and marinate low-cost cuts of beef overnight in above mixture.

Crohn's Disease and IBS:
Enjoy!
Sugar 1 gm; **Fat** 8 gms

Diabetes:
Enjoy!
Carbs 1 gm; **Calories** 82

Heart Disease:
Eliminate the salt and enjoy.
Sodium 32 mgs; **Cholesterol** 0 mgs

LIBBY'S SHISH-KABOB

Ingredients:
1½ pounds lean stew beef
5 cooked carrots, cut in bite size pieces
5 cooked and quartered potatoes
1 green pepper
1 lemon
1 cup barbecue sauce

Temp: Medium
Time: 30 minutes
Yields: 5-6 servings

Directions:
1. Marinate stew beef in beef marinade overnight (see recipe on page 129).
2. Place meat, carrots, green pepper, and potatoes on shish-kabob skewers.
3. Mix lemon juice with barbecue sauce. I use 1 tablespoon per cup of sauce.
4. Cover meat and vegetables with the barbecue mixture and cook over an open grill.
5. Keep basting kabobs with the sauce, until desired tenderness. Delicious!
6. You can use any leftover meat, such as chicken, lamb, etc. with this sauce.

Crohn's Disease and IBS:
Go light on the barbecue sauce.
Sugar 5 gms; **Fat** 6 gms

Diabetes:
Replace the barbecue sauce with one that contains no sugar.
Carbs 35 gms; **Calories** 189

Heart Disease:
Use a low-sodium barbecue sauce, and turkey meat.
Sodium 6 mgs; **Cholesterol** 20 mgs

BENVENUTO'S SPAGHETTI SAUCE AND MEATBALLS

This is my friend Mary's recipe. It came from her family in Italy.
It is my favorite.

Sauce Ingredients:
2 tablespoons extra virgin olive oil
1 onion, chopped
2 cloves garlic
5 (28-ounce) cans crushed tomatoes
1 (15-ounce) can tomato puree
1 small carrot to sweeten
Salt, pepper, and fresh sweet basil to taste
5 sprigs Italian parsley

Temp: Medium
Time: 3 hours
Yields: 8-10 servings

Meatball Ingredients:
2 pounds lean ground beef (98%, plus 3 tablespoons canola oil) or turkey
3 eggs or egg substitute
$1/4$ cup grated low-fat Parmesan cheese
Salt and pepper to taste
1 tablespoon chopped parsley
$3/4$ cup Italian crumbs
1 clove of garlic finely chopped

Directions:
1. Using a large saucepan, brown the onions and cook the garlic in olive oil.
2. When garlic is cooked, remove and throw away.
3. Add crushed tomato puree, carrot, and Italian parsley.
4. Simmer sauce for at least 3 hours.
5. In the meantime, mix all the meatball ingredients together in a food processor.
6. Form meatball mixture into round balls and brown them under the broiler.
7. Add cooked meatballs to sauce the last hour.
8. Serve the sauce and meatballs with your favorite pasta (remove carrots before serving).

Crohn's Disease and IBS:
Use a nondairy Parmesan cheese.
Sugar 10 gms; **Fat** 7 gms

Diabetes:
Replace the Italian crumbs with a gluten-free crumb.
Carbs 21 gms; **Calories** 145

Heart Disease:
Eliminate the salt. Use ground white turkey meat.
Sodium 76 mgs; **Cholesterol** 21 mgs

BARBECUED BEEF SHORT RIBS

Ingredients:
5 pounds beef short ribs (cut into serving pieces)
½ cup canola oil
1 medium onion, chopped
1¼ cups ketchup* or tomato paste
¼ cup brown sugar or Splenda brown sugar blend
¼ cup vinegar
1½ tablespoons low-sodium Worcestershire sauce
2 teaspoons salt
1 teaspoon prepared mustard
1 (8-ounce) package noodles
1 tablespoon all-purpose, unbleached flour (organic)

Ketchup contains some sugar.

Temp: Medium
Time: 2 hours, 20 minutes
Yields: 6 servings

Directions:
1. Braise short ribs on all sides in hot oil.
2. Combine ¾ cup water, onions, ketchup, brown sugar, and vinegar in a bowl; then add the Worcestershire sauce, salt, and mustard.
3. Pour mixture over ribs.
4. Cover pan and simmer 2 hours or until fork tender. Drain, skim off excess fat, and place on heated platter.
5. About 20 minutes before ribs are done, prepare noodles as label directs. Pour in ice water to remove starch in noodles.
6. To thicken sauce, mix 2 tablespoons water with 1 tablespoon flour; stir into sauce and cook, stirring constantly until thickened.
7. Serve sauce over ribs and noodles.

Crohn's Disease and IBS:
Fine to eat. Use Splenda brown sugar blend.
Sugar 20 gms; **Fat** 35 gms

Diabetes:
Use brown rice noodles. Replace ketchup with tomato paste. Use rice flour, and Splenda brown sugar blend.
Carbs 25 gms; **Calories** 149

Heart Disease:
Eliminate the salt. Use the tomato paste in place of ketchup.
Sodium 100 mgs; **Cholesterol** 50 mgs

QUICK AND EASY POT ROAST AND GRAVY

***Perfect if you are in a hurry and want it to look
like you have worked hard on dinner.***

Ingredients:
4 pounds chuck roast
1 can of low-sodium, low-fat cream of mushroom soup
1 package dry onion soup
1 cup of water

Temp: 325° until tender
Time: 3 hours
Yields: 5+ servings

Directions:
1. Place chuck roast in a roasting pan.
2. Pour cream of mushroom soup and dry onion soup on top of roast. Add 1 cup of water.
3. Cover tightly, put in the oven and cook until tender. It makes its own gravy. It cooks itself and tastes wonderful!

Hint: Vegetables may be added to this roast. (Example: potatoes, carrots, onions)

Crohn's Disease and IBS:
Not recommended.
Sugar 2 gms; **Fat** 44 gms

Diabetes:
Use low-fat, low-sodium, dry onion soup. Read the label.
Carbs 3.5 gms; **Calories** 74

Heart Disease:
Use a no sodium cream of mushroom soup, and dry onion soup. Enjoy.
Sodium 95 mgs; **Cholesterol** 128 mgs

HAMBURGER BEEF STROGANOFF

Ingredients:
1 small chopped onion
1 pound 93% lean ground beef (98%, plus 2 tablespoons canola oil)
1 can low-sodium cream of mushroom soup
½ cup low-fat sour cream or low-fat yogurt
Pepper to taste
Canola oil

Temp: Medium
Time: 20 minutes
Yields: 4+ servings

Directions:
1. Sauté onion in cooking oil.
2. Mix beef and canola oil and add to the cooked onions.
3. Stir in cream of mushroom soup.
4. Just before serving add sour cream.
5. Serve over rice or egg noodles.

Crohn's Disease and IBS:
Use a nondairy sour cream and a medium white sauce with mushrooms in place of the cream of mushroom soup.
Sugar 1 gm; **Fat** 1 gm

Diabetes:
Replace the cream of mushroom soup with low-fat cream of mushroom soup. Use rice noodles.
Carbs 3 gms; **Calories** 166

Heart Disease:
Use turkey meat instead of ground beef.
Sodium 87 mgs; **Cholesterol** 55 mgs

MONDAY DISH (English Shepherd's Pie)

Temp: 350°
Time: 25 minutes
Yields: Depends on amount of leftovers

Ingredients:
Leftover meat and gravy
Whipped potatoes

Directions:
1. Place leftover meat and gravy in the bottom of a baking dish.
2. Cover with whipped potatoes.
3. Bake.

Crohn's Disease and IBS:
Use nondairy milk when mashing the potatoes.
Sugar 4 gms; **Fat** 10 gms

Diabetes:
Use skim milk when mashing the potatoes.
Carbs 7 gms; **Calories** 110

Heart Disease:
Make sure the gravy has been put in the refrigerator and the fat has been removed.
Sodium 68 mgs; **Cholesterol** 33 mgs

WHOLESALE PORK CUT

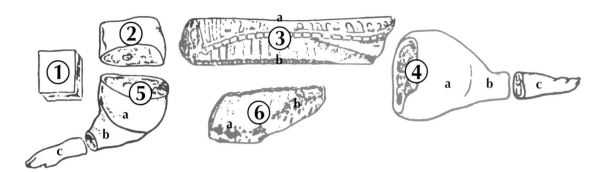

LOW-COST RETAIL CUTS: COLORED BLUE; HIGH-COST RETAIL CUTS: COLORED RED

1. JOWL
Bacon Square

2. SHOULDER BUTT
Rolled Boston Butt
Boston Butt
Blade Steaks
Fresh Shoulder

3. LOIN
a. Fat Back
Salt Pork
Lard
b. Boneless Loin Roast
Bacon
Loin Chops
Rib Chops
Butterfly Chops
Tenderloin
Blade Chops and Roasts
Bacon

4. HAM
a. Smoked Ham Butt Half
b. Smoked Ham Shank Half
(Best Buy) Fresh Ham
c. Back feet (Pig's Feet)

5. PICNIC
a. Fresh Picnic Ham
Smoked Picnic
Canned Luncheon Meat
Armed Roast
b. Fresh Pork Hocks
Smoked Pork Hocks
(for Boiled Dinner)
c. Front Pig's Feet

6. SPARE RIBS
a. Spare Ribs
b. Sliced Bacon
c. Unsliced Bacon

Low-Cost Miscellaneous
- Neck Bone
- Tail
- Kidneys (frozen)
- Liver (frozen)
- Dry Salt Fat Backs
- Fresh Pork Snouts

HINTS

Most pork is a good buy, and is government inspected.

Pork should be properly cooked, because of trichinosis. Fortunately, it has been all but eliminated from modern pork. There were 35 cases of trichinosis reported in 1996. Most were home grown hogs, and wild game.

The government prohibits feeding raw meat and garbage to hogs. Cook fresh pork at 350 degrees until the thermometer registers at 170 degrees. Place the thermometer into the thickest part of the pork or game meat and not near a bone.

Trichinosis is found in wild game products (bear, fox, wolf, horse, seals). Use an accurate meat thermometer as your guide for doneness and safety (if you do eat wild game).

Blade steaks can be used in place of your more expensive loin and rib chops.

Pork is a good source of thiamin. Pork supplies us with three times as much thiamin as other meats. Thiamin helps to steady nerves, promote good digestion and normal appetite.

NEW ENGLAND BOILED DINNER

Some people use corned beef instead of ham in boiled dinners, my family likes ham. My mom used to make boiled dinners when the vegetables were ready for picking. Use 5 pounds of pork hocks if you are on a very strict budget.

Ingredients:
2 pounds whole ham (low-salt, low-fat)
8 small boiling onions
6 medium carrots
3 potatoes
1 turnip
1 teaspoon pepper
1 clove garlic, crushed
1 small cabbage, cut into 6 wedges

Temp: Medium
Time: 1 hour, 15 minutes
Yields: 6 servings

Directions:
1. Place enough water in a large Dutch oven to cover the ham.
2. Sprinkle pepper on the ham and cook for about 1 hour.
3. Next, add the cut up carrots, turnip, small boiling onions, and garlic.
4. Add the cut up potatoes to the other vegetables 10 minutes later (they cook faster).
5. Remove the ham to a platter before adding cabbage.
6. Place the cut up cabbage in the pan, cover and simmer until the cabbage and vegetables are tender, about 15 minutes.
7. Slice the ham and serve with the vegetables.
8. My family likes to add vinegar to the vegetables.

Crohn's Disease and IBS:
Don't eat the turnip or cabbage since they will cause a gassy stomach and are hard to digest.
Sugar 13 gms; **Fat** 22 gms

Diabetes:
Meat consumed should be the size of a deck of cards.
Carbs 16 gms; **Calories** 74

Heart Disease:
Meat consumed should be the size of a deck of cards.
Sodium 89 mgs; **Cholesterol** 34 mgs

RED FLANNEL HASH

Red flannel hash was a great, tasty way to use up the vegetables in the boiled dinner. It's a New England favorite.

Ingredients:
Left over vegetables from the boiled dinner (see recipe on page 138)
1 jar beets
Salt and pepper to taste
Some of the leftover boiled dinner juices

Temp: 350°
Time: ½ hour
Yields: 5 servings

Directions:
1. Finely chop the beets and leftover vegetables.
2. Add salt and pepper and place in a casserole dish with some of the broth from the New England Boiled Dinner.
3. Bake, covered.
4. Serve with slices of leftover ham.

Crohn's Disease and IBS:
Not recommended.
Sugar 5 gms; **Fat** 11 gms

Diabetes:
Eliminate the salt.
Carbs 8 gms; **Calories** 35

Heart Disease:
Eliminate the salt.
Sodium 44 mgs; **Cholesterol** 15 mgs

GLAZED SHOULDER BUTT

Ingredients:
One 3-pound pork shoulder (fat removed)
1 medium onion, sliced
3 whole cloves
1 bay leaf
½ cup brown sugar or Splenda brown sugar blend
1 tablespoon all-purpose, unbleached flour (organic)
½ teaspoon dry mustard
2 tablespoons water

Temp: 350°
Time: Simmer 2 hours, then bake 20 to 30 minutes
Yields: 6-8 servings

Directions:
1. Place pork in deep pan; cover with water.
2. Add onion, cloves and bay leaf. (Put cloves and bay leaf in gauze bag.)
3. Cover tightly; simmer 2 hours. Take out the gauze bag.
4. Remove meat from liquid; place it on rack in shallow roasting pan.
5. Combine brown sugar, flour, mustard, and water.
6. Brush mixture on meat and bake.
7. Remove from oven and let set so the juice will go back through the pork. (Internal temperature should be 170 degrees.)

Crohn's Disease and IBS:
Don't eat any fat. Use a low-fat, low-salt ham.
Sugar 2 gms; **Fat** 60 gms

Diabetes:
Use only 2 teaspoons of brown sugar and rice flour. Use a low-salt, low-fat ham.
Carbs 20 gms; **Calories** 119

Heart Disease:
Use a low-salt, low-fat ham. Have pork loin.
Sodium 39 mgs; **Cholesterol** 11 mgs

ECONOMICAL PORK STEW

Ingredients:
2 tablespoons canola oil
2 medium onions, sliced
1 clove garlic, minced
3 pounds pork stew meat, cut into cubes
1 cup reduced-fat sour cream or low-fat yogurt
$\frac{1}{2}$ teaspoon salt
Pinch of paprika
1 cup water
1$\frac{1}{2}$ cups no yolk egg noodles
$\frac{1}{4}$ cup water
3 tablespoons all-purpose, unbleached flour (organic)

Temp: Low
Time: 1$\frac{1}{2}$ hours
Yields: 6-8 servings

Directions:
1. Lightly brown onion and garlic in canola oil.
2. Push onions and garlic to one side of pan. Add meat and brown.
3. Combine the following ingredients in a small bowl: sour cream, salt, paprika, and one cup of water.
4. Pour mixture over meat.
5. Cover and cook over low heat for 1$\frac{1}{2}$ hours.
6. About 15 minutes before serving, cook noodles as label directs, drain.
7. To thicken gravy mix $\frac{1}{4}$ cup water with 3 tablespoons flour. Gradually add to meat mixture.
8. Serve stew over noodles.

Crohn's Disease and IBS:
Substitute a nondairy sour cream for sour cream.
Sugar 1 gm; **Fat** 10 gms

Diabetes:
Use a rice flour egg noodle (0 mg fat, sodium, cholesterol, wheat, and gluten).
www.ricepasta.com www.tinkyada.com (websites for gluten-free products)
Carbs 13 gms; **Calories** 128

Heart Disease:
Eliminate the salt.
Sodium 9 mgs; **Cholesterol** 100 mgs

PINEAPPLE PORK STEAKS

Ingredients:
4 blade pork steaks
1 (8$\frac{1}{2}$-ounce) can sugar-free sliced pineapple (or fresh)
$\frac{1}{2}$ cup whole cranberry sauce
1 sodium-free, fat-free chicken bouillon cube
$\frac{1}{2}$ cup boiling water
2 tablespoons brown sugar or Splenda brown sugar blend
2 tablespoons vinegar
1 green pepper, cut in 1-inch pieces (optional)
2 tablespoons cornstarch
2 tablespoons water

Temp: Medium to low
Time: 1 hour
Yields: 4 servings

Directions:
1. Trim fat from the steaks.
2. Brown steaks in a frying pan sprayed with cooking spray.
3. Season with salt and pepper.
4. Add the pineapple juice, cranberry sauce, dissolved bouillon cube, brown sugar, and vinegar.
5. Cover and simmer for about 40 minutes.
6. Add the pineapple and green pepper slices in pan and cook for 15 more minutes, covered.
7. Remove steaks and pineapples to a warm platter.
8. Combine cornstarch with 2 tablespoons of water.
9. Stir into cranberry mixture in frying pan.
10. Cook, stirring until thick and bubbly.
11. Pour sauce over steaks.

Crohn's Disease and IBS:
Peel the green pepper and use jellied cranberry sauce. Use only 2 teaspoons brown sugar.
Sugar 13 gms; **Fat** 15 gms

Diabetes:
Eat only 1 ounce lean pork steak, the center loin or loin steak. Add less brown sugar (2 teaspoons). Only buy fresh pineapple with no added sugar.
Carbs 28 gms; **Calories** 216

Heart Disease:
Eliminate the salt and add less brown sugar (2 teaspoons). Only buy fresh pineapple with no added sugar.
Sodium 69 mgs; **Cholesterol** 50 mgs

WHOLESALE LAMB CUTS

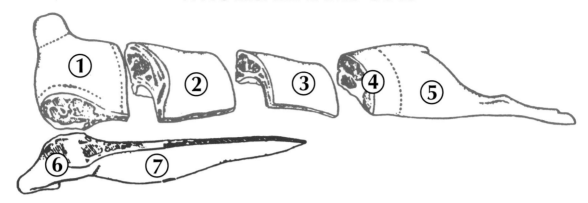

LOW-COST RETAIL CUTS: COLORED BLUE; HIGH-COST RETAIL CUTS: COLORED RED

1. SHOULDER
Saratoga Chops
Shoulder Chops
Blade Chops
Square Cut Shoulder Roast
Lamb Combination, Good Buy

2. RACK
Rack Roast
Rib Chops
Crown Roast

3. LOIN
Loin Chops and Roasts
English Chops

4. SIRLOIN
Sirloin Steaks and Roasts
Cubes for Shish-kabobs

5. LEG
Butt Half
Shank Half (Cost Less)
Boneless rolled leg
Round Steak

6. SHANK
Lamb Shanks

7. BREAST
Lamb Patties
Riblets
Stew Meat
Rolled Breast
Whole Lamb Breast
(make your own spareribs)
Cube Steaks
Flank Steak
Spare Ribs

HINTS

Lamb contains a very small amount of fat and liquid; therefore, cooking it too long will dry it out. It is one of the meats where the flavor lies in the fat.

Mutton comes from an older sheep and is tougher than young sheep. You can tell the difference between mutton and lamb by the bone – lamb has a smooth break while mutton has a jagged break.

Serve lamb either very hot or very cold, never lukewarm, it will taste better.

ROAST LAMB SHANKS

Ingredients:
5 lamb shanks
2 tomatoes, quartered
½ teaspoon salt
1 teaspoon pepper
1 teaspoon paprika
2 cups hot water
5 small potatoes, pared

Temp: 350°
Time: 2 hours
Yields: 5 servings

Directions:
1. Wash lamb shanks.
2. Arrange in open casserole dish.
3. Add tomatoes, salt, pepper, paprika, and water.
4. Cook in a moderate oven - 350° for 30 minutes.
5. Turn meat over and cook another 30 minutes.
6. Add potatoes and cook 30 more minutes.
7. Turn meat and potatoes and cook an additional 30 minutes.
   Total Time: 2 hours.

Crohn's Disease and IBS:
Enjoy! Peel the tomatoes.
Sugar 1 gm; **Fat** 6 gms

Diabetes:
Practice portion control. Enjoy.
Carbs 12 gms; **Calories** 227

Heart Disease:
Eliminate salt.
Sodium 70 mgs; **Cholesterol** 80 mgs

LAMB SHANKS WITH POTATOES AND CARROTS

Ingredients:
4 lamb shanks
¼ cup all-purpose, unbleached flour (organic)
¼ teaspoon salt
⅛ teaspoon pepper
2 tablespoons canola spray
1 small onion, sliced
1¼ cup tomato juice
Pinch oregano
4-6 medium potatoes, pared
4-8 medium carrots

Temp: 350°
Time: 2 hours
Yields: 4 servings

Directions:
1. Coat shanks with flour, salt, and pepper.
2. Brown shanks on all sides in oil in a nonstick frying pan.
3. Transfer meat to large casserole. Sauté cut up onion in frying pan.
4. Combine tomato juice, onion, ½ teaspoon salt, and oregano.
5. Heat to boiling point and pour over shanks.
6. Cover and cook at 350° for 1½ hours.
7. Skim off excessive fat.
8. Add potatoes and carrots.
9. Cook until tender ½ hour longer.

Crohn's Disease and IBS:
Go light on the oregano.
Sugar 9 gms; **Fat** 41 gms

Diabetes:
Use low-sodium tomato juice and rice flour.
Carbs 42 gms; **Calories** 282

Heart Disease:
Eliminate the salt and use a low-sodium tomato juice.
Sodium 66 mgs; **Cholesterol** 59 mgs

LAMB TENDERLOIN WITH PINEAPPLE SAUCE

Ingredients:
6 pounds lamb tenderloin
Salt and pepper to taste
1 (13½-ounce) can sugar-free pineapple chunks
¼ cup pure honey
1 tablespoon balsamic or red wine vinegar
1 teaspoon low-sodium Worcestershire sauce
¼ teaspoon ginger

Temp: 325°
Time: 2 hours, 10 minutes
Yields: 6-8 servings

Directions:
1. Cut tenderloin into serving size pieces.
2. Place tenderloin pieces on racks in a large shallow, open roasting pan.
3. Sprinkle lightly with salt and pepper. Bake for 1½ hours.
4. Meanwhile, make sauce. In a small bowl, drain juice from pineapple (save pineapple). Stir in honey, vinegar, 1 teaspoon salt, Worcestershire sauce and ginger.
5. Remove pan from oven, place tenderloin pieces on a platter. Remove rack and discard drippings.
6. Return tenderloin pieces to pan, cover with sauce and bake 40 minutes, turn meat occasionally.
7. Add pineapple chunks during last 10 minutes.

Crohn's Disease and IBS:
Enjoy, the ginger will help to settle your stomach.
Sugar 11 gms; **Fat** 10 gms

Diabetes:
Eliminate the salt. Enjoy!
Carbs 8 gms; **Calories** 101

Heart Disease:
Eliminate the salt. Enjoy!
Sodium 39 mgs; **Cholesterol** 36 mgs

LAMB STEW

Ingredients:
2 pounds lamb stew meat
(the shank contains less fat than the breast)
4 cups hot water
3 carrots, cut in half
1 small turnip, cut up
1 onion, sliced
2 cups quartered potatoes
2 teaspoons salt
$1/4$ teaspoon pepper
1 bay leaf

Temp: Medium to low
Time: 2$1/2$ hours
Yields: 6 servings

Directions:
1. Flour meat and then brown in a Dutch oven.
2. Add hot water and simmer covered for 2 hours.
3. Add remaining ingredients.
4. Continue cooking until vegetables are tender, about $1/2$ hour.
5. Thicken broth with $1/4$ cup Wondra flour mixed with $1/2$ cup water.
6. Serve with biscuits. (see recipe on page 85)

Crohn's Disease and IBS:
Eliminate the turnip, it's hard to digest and will cause gas.
Sugar 3 gms; **Fat** 8 gms

Diabetes:
Use meat from the shank.
Carbs 14 gms; **Calories** 227

Heart Disease:
Eliminate the salt.
Sodium 81 mgs; **Cholesterol** 76 mgs

LAMB PINWHEELS

Ingredients:
½ pound ground lamb
1 (2-ounce) can chopped mushrooms (packaged in water), drained
2 tablespoons finely chopped onions
1 tablespoon sweet pickle relish
1 tablespoon parsley
1½ cups sifted all-purpose, unbleached flour (organic)
1½ teaspoons baking powder (aluminum-free)
½ teaspoon salt
¼ teaspoon ground sage
¼ cup shortening
½ cup low-fat milk
Gravy (see recipe below)

Temp: 425°
Time: 30 minutes
Yields: 4-6 servings

Directions:
1. Combine lamb, mushrooms, onions, salt, and pepper.
2. Cover and cook 10 minutes over medium low heat, stirring occasionally.
3. Spoon off excess pan juices. Set aside to be used later.
4. Sift flour, baking powder, salt, and sage.
5. Using a pastry blender, cut in shortening until it has the texture of sand.
6. Add milk all at once and stir until blended.
7. Roll out pastry until dough forms a 10″ x 7″ rectangle.
8. Spread meat mixture over dough in an even layer.
9. Start at narrow end, roll jellyroll style.
10. Place seam side down on lightly greased baking sheet.
11. Bake until pastry is lightly browned.

Gravy:
1. Cook 2 tablespoons chopped onions in 2 tablespoons light margarine until tender.
2. Blend in 2 tablespoons flour.
3. Add 1 (10½-ounce) can condensed beef broth.
4. Cook until mixture is thick; season with salt and pepper.
5. Serve over slices of meat roll.

Crohn's Disease and IBS:
Use a nondairy milk in the crust.
Sugar 2 gms; **Fat** 12 gms

Diabetes:
Use lean ground lamb.
Carbs 1 gm; **Calories** 88

Heart Disease:
Eliminate the salt. Use lean ground lamb.
Sodium 71 mgs; **Cholesterol** 94 mgs

POULTRY

Why eat poultry?

I can still smell the turkey roasting in my grandmother's old black stove. All of our family and friends would gather at Nana's to celebrate Thanksgiving and Christmas together. Everyone would bring their favorite dish to be enjoyed by all. Those precious memories will be with me forever. As a child, the aroma of the turkey and its fixings was on my mind, not the fact that the turkey was so good for you.

Poultry is high in protein and low in fat. The dark meat contains more fat than the white meat. Poultry contains all the essential amino acids and is a good source of vitamin B. Dark meat is higher in riboflavin and thiamin, whereas, the white meat is higher in niacin. Turkey is lower in fat than chicken. Only buy free-range, hormone- and antibiotic-free chickens.

Today I'm following the same tradition with my own family and friends – minus the old black stove.

SHOPPING HINTS
1. Buy a whole chicken or turkey and cut it up yourself.
2. If buying separately, poultry wings and legs cost less than the breast per pound.
3. Turkeys are usually a good buy at any time of the year, especially just after Thanksgiving and Christmas.
4. There are always turkey sales in January. A 16-24 pound is your best buy. Less than 10 and over 30 pounds cost the most. Allow $1/2$ pound per person.
5. How you plan on cooking your chicken will determine what kind you will buy. Your stewing hen is an older bird and not very tender. Long, slow, moist cooking will help to tenderize the hen, and make an economical tasty meal.
6. If buying poultry in the summer, place in a cooler with ice when driving home from the grocery store. Bacteria grows rapidly in poultry.

STORAGE
1. Fresh poultry should be loosely wrapped and stored in the refrigerator.
2. It is not wise to refrigerate poultry, or any meat in the original plastic – covered container you receive from the grocery store.
3. Poultry has a tendency to spoil quickly, so plan on using it as soon as possible (within a few days).
4. Poultry may be re-wrapped in freezer paper and frozen. It may be safely stored in the freezer for 6-8 months (whole chickens for 12 months).
5. When freezing, wash poultry in cold water and pat dry. Store in proper freezer bag or foil. Make sure you squeeze out all the air.
6. When thawing poultry, do it in the refrigerator or in cold water…never on the counter top.
7. Cooked turkey in liquid freezes better than dry turkey.
8. Stuffing should be stored separately. Never store the leftover poultry and stuffing together. Don't leave leftover stuffing inside the bird because bacteria will grow.

HOW TO ROAST A DELICIOUS TURKEY OR CHICKEN

1. Place turkey or chicken in the refrigerator to thaw.
2. Remove giblets, etc. located in the body or inside neck cavity.
3. Wash poultry in cold water and pat dry.
4. Season inside of bird.
5. Prepare favorite stuffing.
6. If you choose to stuff poultry, do so just before roasting.
7. Bacteria is high in poultry, so don't leave stuffing in bird. And make sure the stuffing is cold.
8. Fill the neck cavity first. Fold neck skin over and secure with a skewer.
9. Lift up wing tips forcing them back towards the neck shin. It will act as a stand to hold the bird upright.
10. Stuff the body cavity only $^2/_3$ full, stuffing expands.
11. Next, close the cavity opening with small skewers or needle and thread.
12. Press the legs close to the body and tie to tail.
13. Place poultry in a roasting pan breast side up. There are some people that put the breast side down for the first $1^1/_2$ hours, because it takes longer for the dark meat to cook than the white. This way the white breast meat isn't dry or overcooked.
14. Rub margarine over the bird.
15. Place a meat thermometer into the poultry breast. Don't hit the bone.
16. DO NOT ADD WATER!
17. Cook:

Weight	Temp	Approx Cooking Time
$1^1/_2$ to 2 pounds	400°	1 to $1^1/_4$ hours
$2^1/_2$ to 3 pounds	375°	$1^1/_4$ to $1^1/_2$ hours
3 to 4 pounds	375°	$1^1/_2$ to 2 hours
4 to 5 pounds	375°	2 to $2^1/_2$ hours
6 to 7 pounds	375°	$2^1/_2$ to 3 hours
8 to 10 pounds	325°	3 to $3^1/_2$ hours
10 to 14 pounds	325°	$3^1/_2$ to 4 hours
14 to 18 pounds	300°	4 to $4^1/_2$ hours
18 to 20 pounds	300°	$4^1/_2$ to 6 hours

18. Remove bird from oven when cooked. Let it set for 15 to 20 minutes before it is carved. This will insure a moist bird, as the juices will be absorbed back into the bird.
19. Never leave the stuffing inside the bird when storing.
20. Always store stuffing and bird separately to avoid bacterial growth.

Hint: Always wash all poultry thoroughly in cold water to prevent bacteria from growing. Wash counters and cutting boards with disinfectant to prevent cross contamination.

TURKEY CHEDDAR CASSEROLE

Ingredients:

4 ounces broad noodles, cooked
2½ cups diced, cooked turkey
1 (4½-ounce) jar whole mushrooms (optional)
1 tablespoon minced onion
1 cup low-fat milk (or can be liquefied nonfat dry milk)
1 can sodium-free condensed cheese soup
1 cup finely crushed reduced-fat cheese crackers
3 tablespoons melted Smart Balance or another trans fat-free margarine

Temp: 350°
Time: 35 minutes
Yields: 8 servings

Directions:

1. Place noodles in a greased 2-quart casserole.
2. Top with turkey and mushrooms.
3. Blend together onions, milk, and soup.
4. Pour over turkey mixture.
5. Combine cracker crumbs and margarine. Sprinkle over casserole.
6. Bake.

Crohn's Disease and IBS:
Substitute milk with nondairy milk. Make a medium white sauce in place of the cheese soup. Add ½ cup nondairy cheese to the white sauce.
Sugar 3 gms; **Fat** 2 gms

Diabetes:
Substitute rice noodles for flour noodles.
Carbs 8 gm; **Calories** 119

Heart Disease:
Enjoy.
Sodium 92 mgs; **Cholesterol** 19 mgs

TURKEY HASH

Ingredients:
½ cup chopped onion
2 tablespoons canola oil
2 cups diced leftover cooked turkey
¼ cup turkey stock
1 teaspoon salt
½ teaspoon pepper
1 cup diced uncooked potatoes

Temp: Cook over low heat
Time: 10 minutes
Yields: 4 servings

Directions:
1. Sauté onions in oil until brown (10 minutes).
2. Add turkey, stock, salt, and potatoes.
3. Mix well.
4. Cook over low to medium heat 10 minutes.
5. Serve hot.

❖

Crohn's Disease and IBS:
Use canola oil in place of butter or margarine.
Sugar 2 gms; **Fat** 5 gms

Diabetes:
Use canola oil in place of butter.
Carbs 17 gm; **Calories** 210

Heart Disease:
Substitute salt with a pinch of poultry seasoning.
Sodium 42 mgs; **Cholesterol** 87 mgs

TURKEY SHEPHERD'S PIE

Ingredients:
2 cups leftover turkey
2 cups leftover turkey stuffing
½ cup frozen or canned peas
½ cup leftover carrots
1¼ cups leftover turkey gravy (leave gravy in the refrigerator overnight, skim off all fat)
2 cups leftover mashed potatoes
¼ cup low-fat milk or yogurt
Pepper and salt to taste
Nonstick cooking oil

Temp: 350°
Time: 20-25 minutes
Yields: 6 servings

Directions:
1. Spray a 9x9 baking dish with nonstick cooking oil.
2. Spread a layer of stuffing in the baking dish.
3. Next, cover stuffing with ½-inch cubes of turkey.
4. Top with carrots, peas, and gravy.
5. Combine mashed potatoes and warm milk.
6. Spread the potato over the gravy. Sprinkle with salt and pepper.
7. Bake.

This pie may be frozen.

Crohn's Disease and IBS:
Eliminate peas, the outer shell is hard to digest. Replace the milk with nondairy milk.
Sugar 3 gms; **Fat** 8 gms

Diabetes:
Make your stuffing with gluten-free bread or crackers. Use skim milk. Eliminate the peas.
Carbs 12 gm; **Calories** 176

Heart Disease:
Eliminate the salt.
Sodium 100 mgs; **Cholesterol** 0 mgs

TURKEY TURNOVERS

Ingredients:

3 tablespoons reduced-fat margarine

3 teaspoons minced onions

3 tablespoons all-purpose, unbleached flour (organic)

2 teaspoons salt

$1/8$ teaspoon pepper

1 cup nonfat milk

2 cups chopped turkey

Temp: 450°
Time: 20 minutes
Yields: 4 servings

Directions:

1. Melt margarine. Add onions and flour. Mix until smooth.
2. Mix seasoning and add the milk. Stir until thick and smooth.
3. Add turkey and cool the mixture.
4. Make pastry. Roll out $1/8$ inch thick, cut into 3-inch squares.
5. Place a round tablespoon of turkey mixture over $1/2$ and fold the other $1/2$ over the filling. Press the other edges together. Cut steam vents in top of crust. Place on ungreased cookie sheet.
6. Bake.

Crohn's Disease and IBS:
Replace milk with nondairy milk or soymilk.
Sugar 3 gms; **Fat** 12 gms

Diabetes:
Use only 1 teaspoon of salt. Always use skim milk.
Carbs 4 gm; **Calories** 260

Heart Disease:
Eliminate the salt and add a pinch of poultry seasoning for flavor.
Sodium 110 mgs; **Cholesterol** 30 mgs

FRANKS IN A BLANKET

Ingredients:
12 slices reduced-fat bread, crust removed
(whole grain would be healthiest choice)
6 split turkey dogs
6 slices of low-fat cheese
2 eggs, beaten
2½ cups nonfat milk
⅛ teaspoon salt
⅛ teaspoon pepper
¼ teaspoon dry mustard
Cooking spray

Temp: 350°
Time: 1 hour
Yields: 6 servings

Directions:
1. In a greased 12x8x2 pan, place 6 slices of bread.
2. Cover with 6 split hot dogs and slices of cheese.
3. Top with remaining slices of bread.
4. Cover with the combined egg, milk mixture. Add salt and pepper.
5. Refrigerate 1 hour.
6. Bake 1 hour at 350°.

Crohn's Disease and IBS:
Replace the milk with nondairy milk. Either eliminate the cheese or use nondairy cheese.
Use egg substitute.
Sugar 4 gms; **Fat** 11 gms

Diabetes:
Use low-fat cheese, gluten-free bread and egg substitute.
Carbs 22 gm; **Calories** 133

Heart Disease:
Replace the eggs with egg substitute or 4 egg whites. Eliminate the salt. Use low-sodium
bread.
Sodium 100 mgs; **Cholesterol** 27 mgs

CHICKEN CACCIATORE

Ingredients:
2½ pounds boneless, skinless chicken breast
1 cup sliced onions
½ cup thinly sliced green pepper
¼ cup canola oil or extra virgin olive oil
1 chopped medium clove garlic
1 (1-pound) can crushed tomato
½ teaspoon crushed oregano or basil
¼ teaspoon parsley
Dash pepper
½ teaspoon salt
¼ pound sliced mushrooms

Temp: Medium heat
Time: 75 minutes
Yields: 5 servings

Directions:
1. Wash, dry, and cut chicken into approximately ½ to 1-inch pieces.
2. Heat oil in a large skillet. Cook chicken pieces until brown, about 15 minutes.
3. Remove chicken and set aside.
4. Add onion, green pepper, garlic, mushrooms, and cook until onion and peppers are tender.
5. Add crushed tomato, parsley, and spices. Cook over low heat.
6. Add chicken, cover and cook over low heat until all ingredients are tender and hot, about 45 minutes.
7. Stir occasionally.
8. Cook uncovered 15 minutes or until sauce is a good consistency.
9. Serve over your favorite pasta.

Crohn's Disease and IBS:
Peel the green peppers.
Sugar 4 gms; **Fat** 6 gms

Diabetes:
Eliminate the salt.
Carbs 35 gm; **Calories** 180

Heart Disease:
Eliminate the salt.
Sodium 17 mgs; **Cholesterol** 14 mgs

SUNSHINE CHICKEN

Ingredients:
1²/₃ cups thinly sliced carrots
¹/₄ cup butter flavored spray
¹/₄ cup onion, chopped
1 cup orange juice
1 cup water
1 tablespoon sugar (Splenda)
¹/₂ teaspoon salt
¹/₂ teaspoon poultry seasoning
¹/₈ teaspoon pepper
1¹/₂ cups diced cooked chicken (leftover)
1¹/₃ cups Minute Rice (brown rice is a healthier choice)

Temp: Medium
Time: 14 minutes
Yields: 4-5 servings

Directions:
1. Sauté carrots in butter flavored spray until almost tender, about 5 minutes.
2. Add onions and sauté until browned.
3. Add orange juice, water, sugar, salt, poultry seasoning, and pepper. Bring to a boil.
4. Stir in chicken and rice.
5. Cover and simmer 8 minutes or until rice and carrots are tender.

Crohn's Disease and IBS:
Always use acid-free orange juice.
Sugar 1 gm; **Fat** 2 gms

Diabetes:
Enjoy!
Carbs 6 gms; **Calories** 130

Heart disease:
Eliminate the salt.
Sodium 18 mgs; **Cholesterol** 14 mgs

CHICKEN DELIGHT

A great company dish! This is tender on the inside and crispy on the outside. Delicious! Well worth the effort of making this chicken dish.

Ingredients:
3 large chicken breasts
1 teaspoon salt
$1/4$ teaspoon pepper
1 teaspoon rosemary
1 stalk celery, finely chopped
1 cup onions, sliced
1 cup water

Temp: 350°
Time: 1 hour
Yields: 6 servings

Directions:
1. Place the above ingredients in a baking dish and cover.
2. Bake in a 350° oven for one hour.
3. Remove skin and bones; keep chicken in as large pieces as possible.
4. Strain the remaining liquid and reserve as chicken stock.
5. Dip the chicken pieces into the following batter.

Batter:
1 cup all-purpose, unbleached flour (organic)
$1/2$ teaspoons baking powder (aluminum-free)
$1/4$ teaspoon salt
1 beaten egg yolk
$2/3$ cup low-fat milk
$1/4$ cup salad oil
1 egg white, stiffly beaten

Temp: 375°
Time: 3 minutes
Yields: 6 servings

Directions:
1. Sift dry ingredients.
2. Add egg yolk, milk, and oil.
3. Fold in the egg white.
4. Dip chicken pieces into the batter and brown in hot oil.
5. Finish cooking in a 375° oven.
6. Serve with the following sauce.

continued on next page

Sauce:
³/₄ cup reserved chicken stock (refrigerate to harden any fat, discard the fat)
3 tablespoons all-purpose, unbleached flour (organic)
¹/₂ teaspoon salt
Dash of pepper
³/₄ cup evaporated milk (or light cream)
1 tablespoon lemon juice

Directions:
1. Place evaporated milk and flour together in a covered jar. (Add flour last for a smoother sauce.) Shake well.
2. Pour slowly into the heated chicken stock, stirring constantly.
3. Add the lemon juice. Continue stirring until sauce is thick and smooth.
4. Pour over chicken.

Crohn's Disease and IBS:
Make sauce using a nondairy milk. Use egg whites.
Sugar 3 gms; **Fat** 2 gms

Diabetes:
Enjoy!
Carbs 4 gms; **Calories** 246

Heart Disease:
Eliminate the salt. Use skim milk and egg white.
Sodium 100 mgs; **Cholesterol** 38 mgs

CHICKEN AND VEGETABLE BAKE

Ingredients:
½ cup all-purpose, unbleached flour (organic)
½ teaspoon salt
½ teaspoon pepper
1 teaspoon paprika
2½ to 3½ pound broiler fryer (cut up)
¼ cup canola oil
1 cup whole cooked white onions
½ cup coarsely chopped carrots
1 tablespoon brown sugar or Splenda brown sugar blend
¼ teaspoon ginger
1 cup orange juice

Temp: 350°
Time: 1½ hours
Yields: 6-8 servings

Directions:
1. Combine flour, salt, pepper, and paprika in a paper bag.
2. Add chicken and shake (save 2 tablespoons flour mixture).
3. Brown chicken pieces in cooking oil in heavy skillet.
4. Remove chicken to a 2-quart casserole. Add onions and carrots.
5. Blend the 2 tablespoons flour mixture, brown sugar, and ginger into drippings in skillet. Stir to make a smooth paste.
6. Add orange juice and cook until bubbly.
7. Pour over chicken, cover and bake.

Crohn's Disease and IBS:
Enjoy. Use acid-free orange juice. Use Splenda brown sugar blend.
Sugar 4 gms; **Fat** 5 gms

Diabetes:
Use Splenda brown sugar blend.
Carbs 4.5 gms; **Calories** 118

Heart Disease:
Eliminate the salt. Use Splenda brown sugar blend.
Sodium 34 mgs; **Cholesterol** 69 mgs

CHICKEN AND WHIPPED POTATO PIE

Ingredients:
2 cups potatoes (boiled and whipped)
2 tablespoons butter or reduced-fat margarine (Smart Balance)
2 beaten eggs or 4 egg whites
2 tablespoons nonfat milk
$\frac{1}{2}$ teaspoon salt
$\frac{1}{8}$ teaspoon pepper
Chicken in gravy (leftovers)
1 cup peas

Temp: 350°
Time: 1½ hours
Yields: 4 servings

Directions:
1. Combine the potatoes, margarine, eggs, milk, salt, and pepper.
2. Heat the chicken in gravy.
3. Add the peas to the chicken in gravy.
4. Line a buttered pie plate with the whipped potato mixture. Leave a cavity in the center to be filled later with chicken in white sauce or gravy and peas.
5. Brown the potatoes and add the chicken and gravy to the center.
6. Serve.

Crohn's Disease and IBS:
Replace milk with nondairy or soymilk. Replace egg with egg substitute. Eliminate peas.
Sugar 5 gms; **Fat** 4 gms

Diabetes:
Use reduced-fat margarine (Smart Balance). Eliminate peas (they contain sugar).
Carbs 25 gms; **Calories** 193

Heart Disease:
Substitute butter with a heart-safe margarine. Replace the eggs with egg substitute.
Sodium 56 mgs; **Cholesterol** 18 mgs

COMPANY CASSEROLE

Ingredients:
4½-5 pounds ready-to-cook chicken
6 cups water
⅓ cup onion, minced
6 cups medium no-yolk noodles, cooked
1 can condensed low-fat, low-sodium cream of mushroom soup
1½ cups grated low-fat cheddar cheese
1 cup cooked baby peas (leftover)
½ teaspoon salt
¼ teaspoon pepper
Low-fat Parmesan cheese

Temp: 350°
Time: 1 hour, 20 minutes
Yields: 6 servings

Directions:
1. Place chicken in Dutch oven or large pot.
2. Add salt. Cover and cook 2 hours, or until tender.
3. Remove chicken and cut meat into large pieces. Discard bones.
4. Cool broth and skim off any fat. Then add enough water to broth to make 6 cups.
5. Add cooked, drained noodles, soup, cheese, peas, salt, and pepper.
6. In a 3-quart casserole dish, arrange one layer of chicken, another of noodle mixture, repeat, and end with noodles, sprinkled with Parmesan cheese.
7. May be topped with olives around edge.
8. Bake.

May be frozen.

Crohn's Disease and IBS:
Make a medium white sauce and add chopped mushrooms to replace the cream of mushroom. Substitute nondairy cheese for the cheddar cheese. Eliminate the peas.
Sugar 4 gms; **Fat** 21 gms

Diabetes:
Select a gluten-free, low-sodium noodle. Use a sodium-free soup. Eliminate the peas.
Carbs 12 gms; **Calories** 100

Heart Disease:
Eliminate the salt and use a sodium-free soup.
Sodium 137 mgs; **Cholesterol** 74 mgs

CHICKEN NUGGETS

Ingredients:
2 chicken breast fillets
1 egg or 2 egg whites
1 tablespoon canola oil
$\frac{1}{2}$ cup flavored bread crumbs (recipe on page 102)
2 carrots
2 celery stalks

Temp: 350°
Time: 15–20 minutes
Yields: 4-5 servings

Directions:
1. Cut chicken into $1\frac{1}{2}$-inch cubes.
2. In a shallow bowl, whisk together egg and oil.
3. Place breadcrumbs on a separate plate (I use a paper plate, then discard).
4. Dip each chicken piece separately in the egg mixture, then in the breadcrumbs to coat. Pat gently to help crumbs to stick.
5. Place chicken pieces on a nonstick cookie sheet.
6. Bake until juices run clear.
7. Serve with cut up carrots and celery stalk.
8. Make dipping sauce to serve with chicken nuggets. (see pages 164-166)

Crohn's Disease and IBS:
Eliminate the raw carrot and celery sticks. Use egg whites in place of whole eggs.
Sugar 2 gms; **Fat** 7 gms

Diabetes:
Use plain breadcrumbs.
Carbs 16 gms; **Calories** 159

Heart Disease:
Select the egg whites and plain breadcrumbs.
Sodium 109 mgs; **Cholesterol** 59 mgs

BBQ SAUCE

Ingredients:
½ cup organic ketchup (low-sodium)
2 tablespoons brown sugar or Splenda brown sugar blend
1 tablespoon prepared mustard
1 tablespoon water
1 teaspoon low-sodium Worcestershire sauce
¼ teaspoon garlic powder

Temp: Medium to low
Time: 2 or more minutes
Yields: 1 cup

Directions:
1. In saucepan, stir together ingredients.
2. Cook 2 minutes over medium heat, stirring constantly.

Crohn's Disease and IBS: Use milder mustard.
Sugar 6 gms; **Fat** 9 gms

Diabetes: Use 2 teaspoons brown sugar. Ketchup contains some sugar.
Carbs 6 gms; **Calories** 37

Heart Disease: Use 2 teaspoons brown sugar.
Sodium 51 mgs; **Cholesterol** 0 mgs

ORANGE HONEY SAUCE

Ingredients:
½ cup orange juice
2 tablespoons honey
1 tablespoon low-sodium no MSG soy sauce
2 teaspoons cornstarch

Temp: Medium to low
Time: 2 or more minutes
Yields: 1 cup

Directions:
1. In saucepan, stir together ingredients.
2. Cook over medium heat, stirring, until thick and bubbly.

Crohn's Disease and IBS: Use low-acid orange juice and Splenda brown sugar blend.
Sugar 6 gms; **Fat** 0 gms

Diabetes: Use a low-sodium soy sauce, and only 1 tablespoon honey.
Carbs 10 gms; **Calories** 45

Heart Disease: Use a low-sodium soy sauce and only 1 tablespoon of honey. Use Splenda brown sugar blend.
Sodium 1 mg; **Cholesterol** 0 mgs

continued on next page

HOT MUSTARD SAUCE

Ingredients:
¼ cup dry mustard
2 teaspoons canola oil
¼ teaspoon salt
¼ cup hot water

Temp: Medium to low
Time: 2 or more minutes
Yields: 1 cup

Directions:
1. Mix mustard, oil, and salt in a small bowl.
2. Stir in the hot water and mix until blended.

Crohn's Disease and IBS: Enjoy!
Sugar 0 gms; **Fat** 1 gm

Diabetes: Enjoy!
Carbs 0 gms; **Calories** 19

Heart Disease: Eliminate the salt.
Sodium 0 mgs; **Cholesterol** 0 mgs

SWEET AND SOUR SAUCE

Ingredients:
¼ cup brown sugar or Splenda brown sugar blend
1½ teaspoons cornstarch
2 tablespoons red wine vinegar
2 tablespoons pineapple juice (unsweetened)
1½ teaspoons low-sodium soy sauce

Temp: Medium to low
Time: 2 or more minutes
Yields: 1 cup

Directions:
1. Combine brown sugar and cornstarch in a saucepan.
2. Stir in other ingredients.
3. Cook over medium heat, stirring, until thick and bubbly.

Crohn's Disease and IBS: Use Splenda brown sugar blend.
Sugar 7 gms; **Fat** 2 gms

Diabetes: Use unsweetened pineapple juice.
Carbs 8 gms; **Calories** 49

Heart Disease: Use Splenda brown sugar blend.
Sodium 4 mgs; **Cholesterol** 4 mgs

continued on next page

RANCH SAUCE

Ingredients:
½ cup low-fat mayonnaise made with canola oil
¼ cup plain low-fat yogurt
2 teaspoons Parmesan cheese
1 pinch garlic powder
2 tablespoons low-fat milk

Temp: Medium to low
Time: 2 or more minutes
Yields: 1 cup

Directions:
1. Stir mayonnaise and yogurt together in a small bowl.
2. Stir in the cheese, garlic powder, and milk until smooth.

Crohn's Disease and IBS:
Not recommended.
Sugar 1 gm; **Fat** 1 gm

Diabetes:
Use part-skim Parmesan cheese.
Carbs 2 gms; **Calories** 44

Heart Disease:
Use part-skim Parmesan cheese.
Sodium 20 mgs; **Cholesterol** 2 mgs

APRICOT CHICKEN

Ingredients:
1 cup low-sugar apricot jam
1 teaspoon curry powder
1 large chicken, cut in pieces
$\frac{1}{2}$ teaspoon salt
$\frac{1}{2}$ teaspoon pepper
2 medium tomatoes, cut into quarters

Temp: Broil
Time: 27 minutes
Yields: 6 servings

Directions:
1. Mix jam and curry powder in a bowl.
2. Microwave 45 seconds to thin consistency.
3. Sprinkle salt and pepper on chicken.
4. Place chicken under the broiler and cook for 15 minutes.
5. Turn breast sides up and add tomatoes.
6. Broil for additional 10 minutes.
7. Brush chicken and tomatoes with jam mixture.
8. Broil for 2 minutes more, until heated through.

Crohn's Disease and IBS:
Eliminate the curry powder. Use cooked fresh apricots.
Sugar 5 gms; **Fat** 1 gm

Diabetes:
Cook up some fresh apricots with no sugar.
Carbs 7 gms; **Calories** 129

Heart Disease:
Eliminate the salt and use cooked fresh apricots with no sugar.
Sodium 31 mgs; **Cholesterol** 24 mgs

CHICKEN RAGU

Ingredients:
1 (4½-5 pound) roasting chicken (I use a cooked rotisserie
   chicken, it's quick and easy.)
1 medium chopped onion
1 carrot
1 celery stalk
½ to 1 chicken bouillon cube
4 cups water (enough to cover chicken)
Wondra flour and water to thicken the gravy (equal parts)
Salt and pepper to taste

Temp: Medium heat
Time: 2 hours
Yields: 6 servings

Directions:
1. Place the cooked chicken in a heavy, covered pot.
2. Pour 4 cups of water over the chicken.
3. Add a chopped, medium onion, carrot, celery stalk, and chicken bouillon cube to the pot.
4. Cover and cook for 2 hours or until chicken falls off the bone.
5. Remove chicken and set aside. Strain all remaining solids from the pot and discard.
6. Place clear broth back into the pot.
7. Cool chicken and discard all bones and skin. Add salt and pepper.
8. Place pieces of chicken back into the broth.
9. Thicken the broth with a combination of ½ cup Wondra flour, to ½ cup water.
10. Serve hot over mashed potatoes.

Crohn's Diease and IBS:
Use only ½ the chicken bouillon cube.
Sugar 0 gms; **Fat** 1 gm

Diabetes:
Use only ½ the chicken bouillon cube. Omit the salt.
Carbs 2 gms; **Calories** 55

Heart Disease:
Use only ¼ the chicken bouillon cube. Omit the salt.
Sodium 32 mgs; **Cholesterol** 24 mgs

FISH

Why eat fish?

Fish has become increasingly popular in recent years because of taste, health and convenience reasons. Most types of fish are quick and easy to prepare.

Fish is an excellent source of protein, vitamin A, and iron. It's low in fat and is found on many weight watchers diets.

Salt-water fish provide us with iodine. Iodine helps to keep thyroid gland functioning properly. Lack of iodine causes a condition known as Goiter.

Salmon, tuna and sardines are a high source of omega 3 oil, which is considered to be essential for a healthy heart. Cold water salmon is considered by many to be one of the healthiest fish to eat. I personally like it with a raspberry sauce. The recipe is in this chapter.

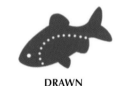   

| DRAWN | DRESSED | STEAK | FILLET |

LOW-COST RETAIL CUTS: COLORED BLUE; HIGH-COST RETAIL CUTS: COLORED RED

Fresh fish can be purchased as drawn, pan dressed, steaks or fillets. The most important issue when buying fresh fish is that the fish is absolutely as fresh as you can obtain.

Drawn fish means the fish is whole except the internal organs have been removed.

Dressed means the fish has been eviscerated and scaled if necessary. Often the head and fins have been removed and the fish is ready to cook.

Drawn and dressed are less expensive than the steak and fillet cuts.

Steaks are cross section slices of large dressed fish such as salmon or halibut. A piece of the backbone is usually still present in the steak, but easily removed after cooking.

Fillets are the strips of flesh from the sides of fish. They are boneless and may still have the skin on one side. The fish dealer will usually remove this skin for you if asked.

Do not hesitate to ask the fish dealer to allow you to smell the fish before purchase. It should smell fresh and mild, with no strong fish smell. If the head is present on the fish, the eyes should be clear and bulging; the gills should be reddish and the scales very shiny.

With fillets or steaks the flesh should be shiny and firm; if pressed with your finger it should spring back.

Before cooking any fresh fish, rinse completely in cold running water and pat dry. Fish can be sautéed, grilled, broiled, poached, or baked. The cooking method usually reflects the fat content of the fish, but all methods can be used satisfactorily.

The best advice on cooking fish is to use what is called the Canadian Cooking Theory. It was developed by the Canadian Department of Fisheries. This cooking theory claims, a fresh fish should have a total cooking time of 10 minutes for each inch of thickness. The fish is measured at its thickest part.

For example, in grilling a halibut steak that is three quarters of an inch thick, the total cooking time is seven and one-half minutes. (Four minutes on one side, and three and one half minutes on the other side.) If you are sautéing a fillet, which is six tenths of an inch thick, it should be cooked three minutes on each side.

Do not neglect frozen fish in your menus. There are excellent products available, and you can use the Canadian Cooking Theory with them. Don't even bother to defrost the fish. Instead of 10 minutes total cooking time per inch of thickness for the fresh fish, use 20 minutes total cooking time for frozen fish. If you have defrosted the fish use the 10-minute rule.

OILY FISH (broil or bake)

Genuine Bluefish – whole, or drawn	Salmon
Mackerel – whole, drawn, fillet	Fresh Tuna
Trout – drawn, dressed, fillets	Herring
Pickerel	Sardines
Butterfish – bony fish – whole, dressed	Lake Trout

DRYER FISH (boil, steam or bake – if basted with fat)
Cod – whole, fillet, drawn, dressed, steaks
Boston Blue - Pollock
Striped bass – whole, dressed, fillet
Ocean perch
Whole flounder – whole, dressed fillets
Carp – whole, fillets
Whiting – whole, or drawn
Brook trout – whole (catch yourself)
Pollock – drawn, dressed, steaks, fillets
Hake – whole, drawn, dressed, fillets
Smelts – whole
Halibut - Haddock

FROZEN
Spanish mackerel – oily

FISH USED FOR CHOWDERS
Cod
Boston Blue – Pollock

HINTS
Whole fish is your best buy. It can be frozen in water for a just caught taste. Stuffed and baked at a low temperature, fish can be very delicious, as well as economical.

Chunk light tuna and flaked tuna are less expensive than solid packed.

COOKING TECHNIQUES

BAKING (clean, wash, and dry fish)

1. Place fish in greased shallow pan.

2. Salt fish and brush with vegetable oil if fish is a dry fish.

3. Cook in a 400° oven.

4. Cook a whole fish 15 minutes for each pound.

5. Do not overcook!

6. Serve fish on a hot platter.

BROILING

1. Place fish on a greased broiler pan.

2. Set oven to broil.

3. Dip 5 fillets in oil and place, with the skin side down, on the broiler pan.

4. Broil for about 3 minutes. Make sure the fish is 2 to 3 inches from the heat.

5. Pour some melted butter or trans fat-free margarine into 1 teaspoon of lemon juice. Serve over the cooked fish for added flavor.

Dill weed is a good seasoning to use on baked and broiled fish.

STORAGE

Fish spoils very quickly, so if frozen fish becomes thawed, cook it immediately. Wrap fish in moisture-proof paper when storing in the refrigerator. Fish can sometimes have a strong odor, so it might be a good idea to either double wrap it or store it in a tightly sealed container. The container may be washed in baking soda and water when you are finished using it. I find that this works very well to eliminate any strong odors.

Another way to eliminate the fish smell from your house is to place a little poultry seasoning in an ashtray and light it with a match. I got the idea from an old Maine fisherman. It really works!

Freeze whole fish in water. It will taste as if you just caught it.

BAKED STUFFED FISH

Ingredients:
3 or 4 pounds dressed fish (halibut or any dry fish)
1½ teaspoons salt
Cooking spray
Bread or low-sodium Town House crackers for stuffing

Temp: 350°
Time: 40-50 minutes
Yields: 4-5 servings

Directions:
1. Clean, wash, and dry fish.
2. Sprinkle inside and outside of fish with salt.
3. Stuff fish loosely with stuffing. (recipe below)
4. Close openings with small skewers or toothpicks.
5. Place fish in well-greased pan.
6. Use cooking spray – if lean fish.
7. Bake in oven.

Bread or Town House Cracker Stuffing:
2 cups bread crumbs or reduced-fat, reduced-sodium Town House cracker crumbs
2 tablespoons butter or trans fat-free margarine
1 teaspoon poultry seasoning
Garlic, chopped and sautéed
Celery, chopped and sautéed
1 whipped egg white

Directions:
1. Sauté breadcrumbs or crackers in margarine.
2. Add poultry seasoning, chopped garlic and celery.
3. Use whipped egg white to bind stuffing.

Hint: Town House crackers have an excellent flavor for stuffing. Lemon juice may be added to the mixture for additional flavor.

Crohn's Disease and IBS:
Enjoy.
Sugar 2 gms; **Fat** 3 gms

Diabetes:
Use unseasoned breadcrumbs in place of cracker crumbs. Use trans fat-free margarine.
Carbs 0 gms; **Calories** 74

Heart Disease:
Eliminate the salt. Use a heart-safe margarine.
Sodium 75 mgs; **Cholesterol** 30 mgs

OVEN BROILED FISH

Ingredients:
2 pounds dressed brook trout or flounder fillets
1 egg, beaten or 2 egg whites
1 tablespoon low-fat milk
$\frac{1}{2}$ teaspoon salt
Dash of pepper
$\frac{1}{2}$ cup all-purpose, unbleached flour (organic)
Canola oil
2 cups low-sodium bread crumbs (see page 102)

Temp: Medium
Time: 8-12 minutes per side
Yields: 4 servings

Directions:
1. Clean, wash, and dry fish.
2. Combine milk, egg, and seasoning.
3. Mix crumbs and flour.
4. Dip fish in egg mixture, and roll in crumb mixture.
5. Cook under broiler for 8-12 minutes on each side.
6. Drain on absorbent paper.

Crohn's Disease and IBS:
Replace milk with a nondairy or soy milk. Use the 2 egg whites.
Sugar 1 gm; **Fat** 11 gms

Diabetes:
Use unflavored breadcrumbs and unbleached flour. Use the 2 egg whites.
Carbs 5 gms; **Calories** 100

Heart Disease:
Use the egg white and eliminate the salt. Use no sodium crackers.
Sodium 54 mgs; **Cholesterol** 87 mgs

SALMON WITH PECANS

Ingredients:
2 cups pecans (no salt)
1 tablespoon minced garlic
¼ teaspoon ground pepper
½ cup extra virgin olive oil
8 pieces salmon fillets (approximately 4 lbs)

Temp: 450°
Time: 4-5 minutes
Yields: 8 servings

Directions:
1. Grind pecans until fine.
2. Add garlic and pepper, mix with pecans.
3. Brush salmon in olive oil and roll in pecan mix.
4. Sauté salmon on one side.
5. Place salmon on a cookie sheet.
6. Bake for 4-5 minutes.

Crohn's Disease and IBS:
If nuts bother you, use breadcrumbs.
Sugar 2 gms; **Fat** 25 gms

Diabetes:
Have only 6 pecans.
Carbs 6 gms; **Calories** 349

Heart Disease:
Have only 6 pecans or use crushed walnuts.
Sodium 100 mgs; **Cholesterol** 135 mgs

RASPBERRY SAUCE

Wonderful sauce! I first had this raspberry sauce on salmon at my son's wedding reception in California. The combination of the sauce with salmon was superb.

Ingredients:
1 (10-ounce) pkg frozen red raspberries in light syrup, thawed
1 tablespoon cornstarch

Temp: Medium to low
Time: Until thick
Yields: 1 cup

Directions:
1. In a small saucepan, combine raspberries and cornstarch; cook and stir until thickened and clear.
2. Pour sauce onto salmon.

Crohn's Disease and IBS:
Puree and strain the sugar-free raspberries.
Sugar 2 gms; **Fat** 2 gms

Diabetes:
Only use sugar-free frozen raspberries or fresh berries.
Carbs 8 gms; **Calories** 23

Heart Disease:
Use sugar-free raspberries or fresh berries.
Sodium 7 mgs; **Cholesterol** 0 mgs

SALMON ON THE GRILL

Ingredients:
2 tablespoons melted butter or trans fat-free margarine (Smart Balance)
½ teaspoon dill weed
1 lemon
¼ teaspoon onion powder
1 tablespoon pepper
1 pound salmon fillets

Temp: Medium
Time: 15 minutes
Yields: 4 servings

Directions:
1. Place fillets on heavy-duty aluminum foil.
2. Spread mixed butter, dill, onion powder, lemon juice, and pepper over salmon fillets.
3. Cook on grill for 15 minutes, turning after 5-7 minutes.

Crohn's Disease and IBS:
Use Smart Balance or another trans fat-free margarine.
Sugar 0 gms; **Fat** 13 gms

Diabetes:
Use Smart Balance or another trans fat-free margarine.
Carbs 0 gms; **Calories** 138

Heart Disease:
Use Smart Balance or another trans fat-free margarine.
Sodium 102 mgs; **Cholesterol** 104 mgs

LIME AND PARSLEY BAKED SALMON

Ingredients:
1 clove garlic, finely chopped
1 egg or 2 egg whites
1 teaspoon lime juice
$1/2$ teaspoon salt
$1/4$ teaspoon pepper
$1/2$ cup canola oil
$4^1/_2$ teaspoons extra virgin olive oil
4-5 sprigs fresh parsley
2-3 salmon steaks (salmon steaks should be the size of a deck of cards per person)

Temp: 400°
Time: 8-10 minutes
Yields: 4 servings

Directions:
1. Place garlic, egg, lime juice, salt, and pepper in food processor.
2. Add the canola oil and olive oil pouring very slowly (saving just a little to brush on the salmon). It should start to look like mayonnaise.
3. Add chopped parsley (keep blending).
4. Brush salmon with remaining oil, salt, and pepper to taste.
5. Spread sauce over salmon steaks.
6. Bake for 8-10 minutes at 400°.

Crohn's Disease and IBS:
Use 2 egg whites in place of whole egg.
Sugar 1 gms; **Fat** 89 gms

Diabetes:
Use 2 egg whites in place of whole egg.
Carbs 0 gms; **Calories** 490

Heart Disease:
Eliminate the salt and use 2 egg whites in place of whole egg.
Sodium 105 mgs; **Cholesterol** 67 mgs

ROASTED SALMON

Ingredients:
¼ cup sugar-free pineapple juice
2 tablespoons lemon juice
4 (6-ounce) salmon fillets (Alaskan, not farm raised)
2 tablespoons brown sugar or Splenda brown sugar blend
4 teaspoons chili powder
2 teaspoons grated lemon zest
¼ teaspoon salt
¼ teaspoon cinnamon

Temp: 400°
Time: 12 minutes
Yields: 4 servings

Directions:
1. Preheat oven.
2. Combine the first 3 ingredients and marinate in a zip lock bag for 1 hour in the refrigerator.
3. Remove fish from bag and discard marinade.
4. Combine sugar, chili powder, lemon zest, salt, and cinnamon.
5. Rub into salmon fillets.
6. Place in an 11x7 baking dish.
7. Bake for 12 minutes.
8. Serve with lemon wedges and brown rice.

Crohn's Disease and IBS:
Omit the chili powder. Use Splenda brown sugar blend.
Sugar 5 gms; **Fat** 3 gms

Diabetes:
Use Splenda brown sugar blend.
Carbs 11 gms; **Calories** 274

Heart Disease:
Eliminate the salt. Use Splenda brown sugar blend.
Sodium 102 mgs; **Cholesterol** 135 mgs

SALMON LOAF

Ingredients:

1 large (16-ounce) can red salmon (Alaskan)

½ teaspoon salt

¼ teaspoon paprika

¼ teaspoon pepper

3 tablespoons lemon juice

3 egg whites

¼ cup melted butter or trans fat-free Smart Balance margarine

3 egg yolks (substitute 3 more egg whites instead if you are on a low-cholesterol diet)

1½ cups firmly packed soft bread crumbs (whole grain, better choice)

1½ cups scalded nonfat milk

Temp: 350°
Time: 1 hour
Yields: 8 servings

Directions:

1. Remove the bones and skin from the salmon.
2. Mix the salmon with the salt, pepper, paprika, lemon juice, melted butter, beaten egg yolks, and breadcrumbs. Mix thoroughly.
3. Add the warm milk to this mixture.
4. Beat the egg whites until stiff and fold into the batter.
5. Pour the mixture into a greased loaf pan.
6. Bake.
7. Serve with the egg white sauce. (Recipe on the next page.)

Crohn's Disease and IBS:
Use a nondairy milk. Use all egg whites.
Sugar 2 gms; **Fat** 100 gms

Diabetes:
Replace the butter with Smart Balance trans fat-free margarine. Substitute the egg yolks with egg substitute or egg whites. Use a low-carb bread and skim milk.
Carbs 8 gms; **Calories** 10

Heart Disease:
Only use the egg substitute and egg whites. Use low-sodium bread.
Sodium 64 mgs; **Cholesterol** 47 mgs

EGG WHITE SAUCE

Directions:
4 tablespoons reduced-fat margarine
4 tablespoons all-purpose, unbleached flour (organic)
Dash white pepper
$\frac{1}{2}$ teaspoon salt
2 cups reduced-fat milk
2 hard cooked eggs

Temp: Medium heat
Time: 5 minutes
Yields: 8 servings

Directions:
1. Melt the margarine in a saucepan over medium to low heat.
2. Stir the flour into the melted margarine.
3. Then slowly add the milk, stirring constantly.
4. Add the salt and pepper.
5. Cook over a low heat, until the sauce thickens (use a wooden spoon to stir).
6. Thinly slice the hard cooked eggs and add to the sauce.
7. Pour over the salmon loaf.

Crohn's Disease and IBS:
Substitute nondairy milk in place of fat-free milk. Use Smart Balance margarine.
Eliminate the yolk from the hard cooked egg.
Sugar 3 gms; **Fat** 4 gms

Diabetes:
Enjoy. Use Smart Balance margarine and skim milk.
Carbs 3 gms; **Calories** 27

Heart Disease:
Eliminate the yolk from the hard cooked eggs. Eliminate the salt. Use Smart Balance margarine.
Sodium 37 mgs; **Cholesterol** 1 mg

HOMEMADE TARTAR SAUCE

Ingredients:
1 cup low-fat mayonnaise made with canola oil
1 teaspoon grated onion
2 tablespoons minced dill pickles
1 tablespoon minced parsley

Time: 5 minutes
Yields: 1¼ cups

Directions:
1. Combine all the above ingredients.
2. Store in a covered container in the refrigerator.

Crohn's Disease and IBS:
Eat in moderation. Finely chop the dill pickle.
Sugar 1 gm; **Fat** 2 gms

Diabetes:
Use only 1 tablespoon dill pickles.
Carbs 1 gm; **Calories** 49

Heart Disease:
Use only 1 tablespoon dill pickles.
Sodium 50 mgs; **Cholesterol** 10 mgs

SARDINE STUFFED TOMATOES

Sardines are full of omega 3 oil.

Ingredients:

Yields: 4 servings

2 cans sardines (in soybean oil)
1/3 cup diced celery
1 tablespoon diced onions
2 tablespoons reduced-fat salad dressing
2 drops tabasco sauce (optional)
4 small tomatoes

Directions:

1. Open can and save 4 sardines.
2. Drain cans.
3. Add celery, onions, and other ingredients.
4. Mix well.
5. Peel tomatoes and scoop out some of the center.
6. Fill cavity with the sardine mixture.
7. Place whole sardine on top.
8. Serve on bed of lettuce.

Crohn's Disease and IBS:
Not recommended.
Sugar 3 gms; **Fat** 35 gms

Diabetes:
Use reduced-calorie salad dressing.
Carbs 2 gms; **Calories** 62

Heart Disease:
Enjoy. Omega 3 oil is great for your heart. Use low-sodium sardines.
Sodium 39 mgs; **Cholesterol** 30 mgs

ANITA'S CRABMEAT ENGLISH MUFFINS

Ingredients:
½ cup low-fat margarine or butter
1 small jar (5-ounce) Old English cheese spread
½ teaspoon low-sodium Worcestershire sauce
¼ teaspoon garlic powder (not garlic salt)
Pepper to taste
7 ounces canned crabmeat (or fresh), drained
6 100% whole grain English muffins

Temp: Broiler
Time: Until bubbly
Yields: 72 pieces

Directions:
1. Soften and cream together the margarine and cheese.
2. Add the Worcestershire, salt, pepper, and garlic powder.
3. Mix well and add the drained crabmeat.
4. Spread the crabmeat mixture over the English muffin halves.
5. Refrigerate about 1 hour before cutting each half into 6 wedges.
6. Place muffin wedges under the broiler until bubbly and light brown.

Crohn's Disease and IBS:
Use a nondairy cheese spread and trans fat-free margarine. Replace whole grain English muffin with the original English muffin.
Sugar 5 gms; **Fat** 8 gms

Diabetes:
Replace butter with trans fat-free margarine.
Carbs 3 gms; **Calories** 2

Heart Disease:
Use trans fat-free margarine and low-sodium English muffins.
Sodium 30 mgs; **Cholesterol** 1 mg

STUFFED RED SNAPPER

Ingredients:

1 (3-pound) fresh or frozen dressed red snapper or other fish
Nonstick spray coating
³/₄ cup chopped onion
³/₄ cup chopped celery
1 tablespoon light butter or trans fat-free margarine
1¹/₂ cups cooked brown rice or long grain rice
1 cup chopped tomato
¹/₃ cup snipped fresh parsley (or grow your own)
¹/₂ teaspoon dried thyme, crushed

Temp: 350°
Time: 50-60 minutes
Yields: 8 servings

Directions:

1. Thaw fish, if frozen. Rinse fish and pat dry with paper towels. Spray a shallow baking pan with nonstick spray coating.
2. For stuffing, in a skillet cook onion and celery in margarine until vegetables are tender. Stir in rice, tomato, parsley, and thyme. Spoon stuffing into cavity of fish. Do not pack tightly. Tie or skewer the fish to close. Cover loosely with foil.
3. Bake until fish flakes easily when tested with a fork.

Crohn's Disease and IBS:
Use trans fat-free margarine.
Sugar 1 gm; **Fat** 3.6 gms

Diabetes:
Use Smart Balance trans fat-free margarine.
Carbs 8 gms; **Calories** 94

Heart Disease:
Use a heart-safe margarine. (Promise)
Sodium 50 mgs; **Cholesterol** 23 mgs

GAIL'S FETTUCINE ALFREDO with Shrimp, Broccoli, and Mushrooms

Ingredients:
½ pound fettuccine, cooked according to package directions
½ pound broccoli florets
16 ounces soy milk
3 egg yolks or egg substitute
3 tablespoons trans fat-free margarine
2 tablespoons fresh basil, chopped
4 ounces sliced mushrooms
1 pound 26/30 shrimp (frozen less expensive)
1 shallot, minced
1 teaspoon minced garlic
½ cup low-fat Parmesan cheese
½ cup low-fat milk
Salt and pepper to taste

Temp: Medium
Time: 7 minutes
Yields: 6-8 servings

Directions:
1. Peel shrimp and rinse in cold water.
2. Heat 3 tablespoons margarine in sauté pan and sauté shallots, garlic, and mushrooms for 2-3 minutes. Add shrimp and sauté 3-4 minutes.
3. Blanch and shock broccoli florets (cook in a double boiler until tender, then place in cold water).
4. Mix egg yolks with soy milk in a separate bowl.
5. Remove shrimp and vegetables. Pour in milk and yolk mixture, reduce heat to simmer.
6. Add Parmesan cheese and chopped basil.
7. Reduce by ⅓ and add low-fat milk to make desired consistency.
8. Season with salt and pepper.
9. Mix cooked pasta, shrimp/vegetable mixture, and soy milk.
10. Toss to incorporate.

Crohn's Disease and IBS: Replace milk with a nondairy substitute. Replace eggs with an egg substitute. Use soy Parmesan cheese.
Sugar 2 gms; **Fat** 3 gms

Diabetes: Replace milk with skim milk and eggs with an egg substitute.
Carbs 6 gms; **Calories** 68

Heart Disease: Replace milk with skim milk. Eliminate salt. Use an egg substitute.
Sodium 77 mgs; **Cholesterol** 4 mgs

FRESH WATER TROUT

Ingredients:
²/₃ cup bread crumbs (see page 102)
¹/₄ cup all-purpose, unbleached flour (organic)
¹/₂ teaspoon salt
¹/₂ teaspoon pepper
¹/₂ teaspoon paprika
6 trout (approx. ¹/₂ pound each)
Canola oil

Temp: Medium
Time: 4 minutes per side
Yields: 6 servings

Directions:
1. Combine bread crumbs, flour, 1/2 teaspoon salt, pepper and paprika.
2. Coat fish with mixture.*
3. Heat oil in a skillet.
4. Cook fish until lightly browned – 4 minutes on each side.
5. Do not overcook.

May put ingredients with fish into a Ziploc bag and shake.

Crohn's Disease and IBS:
Enjoy!
Sugar 1 gm; **Fat** 3 gms

Diabetes:
Enjoy!
Carbs 1 gm; **Calories** 113

Heart Disease:
Enjoy!
Sodium 58 mgs; **Cholesterol** 29 mgs

BROILED SOLE WITH LEMON AND TOMATO

Ingredients:
2 sole fillets (4 ounces each)
Lemon pepper seasoning to taste
1 firm tomato, finely chopped
1/4 teaspoon crushed dried thyme
1/4 teaspoon garlic powder
1/2 tablespoon lemon juice

Temp: Broil
Time: 6 minutes
Yields: 2 servings

Directions:
1. Rinse the fillets and pat dry using a paper towel.
2. In a small baking dish, place the fish in a single layer.
3. Combine the remaining ingredients in a small bowl.
4. Spoon the mixture evenly onto the fillets.
5. Broil fillets about 4 inches from the broiler unit for 5 or 6 minutes, without turning.
6. The fish should flake easily with a fork.

Crohn's Disease and IBS:
Peel the tomato before cooking and chopping.
Sugar 2 gms; **Fat** 2 gms

Diabetes:
Enjoy!
Carbs 3 gms; **Calories** 141

Heart Disease:
Enjoy!
Sodium 3 mgs; **Cholesterol** 86 mgs

VINALHAVEN CRAB CAKES WITH MY LOBSTER SAUCE

Vinalhaven, Maine is an island about 15 miles east, out to sea, from Rockland, Maine. You have to take the Maine State Ferry to get to the island. The sights to the island are breathtaking. The people are wonderful and make everyone feel at home. Their major economy revolves around lobster fishing. Vinalhaven has the best seafood of any place in New England. I personally like their crab cakes and delicious lobsters. I hope you enjoy these crab cakes with my lobster sauce, I know I do.

Ingredients:
1 cup fresh crabmeat
1 cup mashed potatoes
20 salt-free crackers, finely rolled
1 egg or 2 egg whites
1 tablespoon minced onions
Pinch pepper
Cracker meal (gluten-free)

Temp: Medium to low
Time: Until golden brown
Yields: 8 servings

Directions:
1. Place fish in a fine strainer and run water over it for a few minutes.
2. Blend together crabmeat, potatoes, cracker crumbs, egg, onion, and pepper.
3. Shape into 8 patties; roll in cracker meal.
4. Sauté until golden brown.
5. Good served with lobster sauce. (See recipe on page 189)

Crohn's Disease and IBS:
Use 2 egg whites. Enjoy!
Sugar 1 gm; **Fat** 1 gm

Diabetes:
Use 2 egg whites. Enjoy!
Carbs 9 gms; **Calories** 51

Heart Disease:
Use 2 egg whites. Enjoy!
Sodium 30 mgs; **Cholesterol** 10 mgs

LOBSTER SAUCE

Incidently, have you ever wondered how to tell the difference between the male and female lobster? Who has the most meat? Since the male is territorial and fights, he has larger claws. The female carries her eggs in her tail, which is wider than the males.

Ingredients:
1 cup medium white sauce
1 cup finely cut up lobster meat (114 gms meat)

Temp: Medium to low
Time: 5 minutes
Yields: 8 servings

Medium white sauce:
2 tablespoons Smart Balance margarine
2 tablespoons all-purpose, unbleached flour (organic)
Pinch salt
1 cup low-fat milk

Directions:
1. Make a medium white sauce as follows.
2. Heat margarine in a saucepan over low heat until melted.
3. Blend in the flour, salt, and pepper.
4. Cook over low heat, stirring constantly, until smooth and bubbly.
5. Remove from heat and stir in the milk, stirring constantly. Cook for one minute.
6. Stir in the chopped lobster meat. Serve over the crab cakes.

Lobster contains low-fat, B_{12}, protein, zinc, and omega 3 fatty acid.

Crohn's Disease and IBS:
Substitute nondairy milk for the low-fat milk.
Sugar 4 gms; **Fat** 9 gms

Diabetes:
Substitute with skim milk.
Carbs 16 gms; **Calories** 30

Heart Disease:
Omit salt.
Sodium 42 mgs; **Cholesterol** 18 mgs

MEAT ALTERNATIVES

Why eat meat alternatives?

Legumes, such as dry beans, peas, lentils, and nuts are a secondary source of protein. Soybeans and peanuts are the only two legumes containing a high quality protein. Milk added to the other legumes will give you the necessary high quality protein needed to meet your daily requirements.

Beans are believed to be good for your heart. A study at Tulane University found that those who ate legumes at least four times a week had a 22% lower risk of heart disease than those who ate it once a week. They also had lower blood pressure and LDL (bad) cholesterol.

BUYING LOW COST LEGUMES

Soybeans
Split peas – yellow and green
Pea beans
Kidney beans
Lima beans
Lentils

STORAGE

Store in original containers, in cupboard.

COOKING TECHNIQUES

LENTILS

Lentils are one of the few legumes that may be cooked without soaking. Boil about $\frac{1}{2}$ hour in salt water.

DRY BEANS AND PEAS

Soak beans or peas in cold water overnight. If you forget to soak them, parboil peas or beans in water until the skin wrinkles. Drain beans and place in a bean pot. Combine all your seasonings and stir into the beans. Cover beans with boiling water. Place salt pork on top of beans. Cover bean pot and bake beans at 250° for about 8 hours. Stir occasionally. The last hour or so, uncover bean pot, so the top of beans will brown.

DRIED SOYBEAN CASSEROLE

Ingredients:
2 cups yellow soybeans
2 teaspoons salt
1 small onion
2 tablespoons light brown sugar or Splenda brown sugar blend
2 tablespoons molasses
1 teaspoon prepared mustard
¼ pound Canadian bacon (a better choice than salt pork)

Temp: 250°
Time: 8 hours
Yields: 8 servings

Directions:
1. Soak beans overnight in water in covered container.
2. Drain and cover with fresh water.
3. Heat to boiling and cook until tender, about 3 hours.
4. Mix beans with remaining ingredients; place in greased casserole.
5. Bake casserole in oven at 250° for 5 hours.

Crohn's Disease and IBS:
Not recommended.
Sugar 7.6 gms; **Fat** 5 gms

Diabetes:
Use Splenda brown sugar blend.
Carbs 12 gms; **Calories** 43

Heart Disease:
Eliminate the salt.
Sodium 22 mgs; **Cholesterol** 3 mgs

TOFU AND CORN QUICHE

Ingredients:
1 teaspoon trans fat-free margarine or butter
2 tablespoons fine dry bread crumbs
12 ounces tofu (fresh bean curd), drained
2 egg whites
1 egg
$^1/_3$ cup 1% milk
$^1/_2$ teaspoon dried oregano, crushed
Pinch of garlic powder
$^3/_4$ cup shredded low-fat cheddar cheese
1 (7-ounce) can whole kernel corn with sweet peppers, drained
1 tablespoon dried minced onion
1 medium tomato
1 tablespoon snipped fresh parsley (optional)

Temp: 350°
Time: 30-35 minutes
Yields: 4 servings

Directions:
1. Spread the margarine over the bottom and sides of a greased 9-inch pie plate. Sprinkle with bread crumbs to coat the dish.
2. Cut up tofu.
3. In a blender container or food processor bowl combine tofu, egg whites, whole egg, milk, oregano, garlic powder, $^1/_2$ cup of the cheese, $^1/_4$ teaspoon pepper, and $^1/_8$ teaspoon salt.
4. Cover and blend or process until smooth. Stir in corn and dried onion. Pour into prepared pie plate.
5. Bake, uncovered, until a knife inserted near the center comes out clean.
6. Cut tomato into thin wedges. Arrange wedges on top of the quiche. Sprinkle with the remaining cheese. Bake for 3 minutes more or until cheese is melted.
7. Garnish with fresh parsley, if desired.

Crohn's Disease and IBS:
Not recommended.
Sugar 1 gm; **Fat** 5 gms

Diabetes:
Change the crumbs to gluten-free crumbs. Use low-fat cheese and low-fat skim milk. Corn contains sugar.
Carbs 10 gms; **Calories** 107

Heart Disease:
Replace milk with low-fat skim milk. Use only 4 egg whites. Eliminate salt.
Sodium 49 mgs; **Cholesterol** 0 mgs

YELLOW SPLIT PEA STEW

Ingredients:
1 pound yellow split peas
2 teaspoons salt
Meaty ham bone
4 potatoes, quartered
4 small carrots, cut in half
1 onion, quartered

Temp: Medium to low
Time: 2-3 hours
Yields: 6 servings

Directions:
1. Soak peas in 2 quarts of water overnight.
2. Add salt, pepper, and ham bone.
3. Cook for 2 to 3 hours until peas are soft.
4. Add vegetables the last ½ hour.
5. If the stew needs it add more water.
6. Serve with corn bread for a delicious, nutritious meal.

❖

Crohn's Disease and IBS:
Not recommended.
Sugar 5 gms; **Fat** 2 gms

Diabetes:
Eliminate the salt.
Carbs 15 gms; **Calories** 72

Heart Disease:
Eliminate the salt.
Sodium 8 mgs; **Cholesterol** 2 mgs

BOSTON BAKED BEANS

We had homemade baked beans every Saturday after the matinee movies. There was no better smell than the beans baking all day in my grandmother's black wood stove. Of course as kids, and having seen a cowboy movie, we had to eat our beans out of a tin pan. In the summer, Nana would bake the beans in a special pit built under the ground. Some Maine people still cook them that way today. As kids we loved a baked bean sandwich, nobody could make them as good as Nana.

Ingredients:
2 cups pea beans
1/2 pound salt pork or Canadian bacon
1 sliced onion
3 tablespoons blackstrap molasses
(Spray cup with cooking oil first and the molasses will empty easily.)
2 teaspoons salt
1/8 teaspoon pepper
1/4 teaspoon dry mustard

Temp: 250°
Time: 8 hours
Yields: 6-8 servings

Directions:
1. Soak beans overnight in 1-quart cold water with a teaspoon of baking soda (baking soda prevents gassy stomach).
2. Simmer in same water for about 15 minutes.
3. Drain, rinse, and add fresh water.
4. Place beans, pork, and onion in a bean pot.
5. Combine molasses and seasonings; pour over beans.
6. Cover and bake.

Crohn's Disease and IBS:
Not recommended.
Sugar 5 gms; **Fat** 3 gms

Diabetes:
Make beans with no pork and only 1½ tablespoons of molasses. (Buy the vegetarian style if you don't make your own beans.)
Carbs 17 gms; **Calories** 84

Heart Disease:
Make beans with no salt pork and eliminate the salt.
Sodium 38 mgs; **Cholesterol** 2 mgs

BEANS–N–GREENS

Ingredients:
2 cups dried white beans
8 cups water
2 slices chopped salt pork or Canadian bacon
1 cup chopped onions
2 tablespoons all-purpose, unbleached flour (organic)
2 teaspoons salt
½ teaspoon black pepper
1 bunch escarole, shredded

Temp: Medium to low
Time: 2½ hours
Yields: 6 servings

Directions:
1. Wash beans, cover with water, and bring to a boil. Turn off heat and let soak 1 hour.
2. Drain; add water, bring to a boil, cover and cook over low heat 1½ hours.
3. In large skillet, cook salt pork or bacon, and onions until brown.
4. Blend in flour.
5. Add salt pork or bacon, onions, and flour mixture to beans with salt and pepper.
6. Cook 30 minutes.
7. Add escarole; cook 30 minutes until beans are tender.
8. Taste for seasoning.

Crohn's Disease and IBS:
Not recommended.
Sugar 2 gms; **Fat** 4 gms

Diabetes:
Eliminate the salt pork, use a small piece of Canadian bacon instead. Don't add salt.
Carbs 21 gms; **Calories** 134

Heart Disease:
Eliminate salt and salt pork.
Sodium 45 mgs; **Cholesterol** 4 mgs

MACARONI AND CHEESE CASSEROLE

Ingredients:
1 pound box elbow macaroni (whole grain)
½ pound reduced-fat cheddar cheese, grated
½ pound low-fat Monterey Jack cheese, grated
4 ounces low-fat cream cheese
1 tablespoon trans fat-free margarine
2 whipped egg whites
½ to ¾ cup 1% milk
1 (1 pound) can drained chopped tomatoes
Salt and pepper to taste
¼ cup seasoned bread crumbs (see recipe on page 102)
¼ cup finely ground almonds

Temp: 350°
Time: 45 minutes to 1 hour
Yields: 6-8 servings

Directions:
1. Preheat oven.
2. Cook macaroni according to package directions and drain.
3. Cut cream cheese into cubes.
4. Add margarine, cheeses, eggs, milk, tomatoes, salt and pepper to macaroni, mix well.
5. Pour into a greased 9x13 pan.
6. Mix crumbs and ground almonds together, sprinkle crumbs on top.
7. Bake.

Crohn's Disease and IBS:
Use nondairy cheeses and milk (soy). Eliminate the almonds.
Sugar 0 gms; **Fat** 3 gms

Diabetes:
Use no carb bread for crumbs. Replace milk with skim milk.
Carbs 18 gms; **Calories** 176

Heart Disease:
Eliminate salt. Eat sparingly.
Sodium 125 mgs; **Cholesterol** 2 mgs

BLACK BEAN LASAGNA

Ingredients:
9 lasagna noodles (whole grain, healthier choice)
½ cup chopped onion
½ cup chopped red bell pepper
½ cup frozen corn kernels, thawed (optional – corn is a starchy vegetable)
2 cloves garlic, chopped
1 (15-ounce) can black beans, rinsed and drained
1 (16-ounce) can refried black beans
2¾ cups canned tomato sauce
½ cup salsa
½ cup chopped fresh cilantro, divided
1½ cups fat-free cottage cheese
1 cup fat-free ricotta cheese
¼ cup fat-free sour cream or yogurt
8 ounces fat-free Monterey Jack cheese, shredded
¼ cup sliced ripe olives
8 sprigs fresh parsley

Temp: 350°
Time: 1 hour
Yields: 8 servings

Directions:
1. Preheat oven. Bring a large 5-quart pot of lightly salted water to a boil. Add pasta and cook for 8 to 10 minutes or until al dente; drain.
2. Coat a large skillet with non-stick cooking spray, place over medium heat. Sauté onion, red bell pepper, corn, and garlic until tender. Stir in black beans, refried beans, tomato sauce, salsa, and ¼ cup cilantro. Cook until heated through and slightly thickened; set aside.
3. In a large bowl, combine cottage cheese, ricotta, sour cream, shredded Monterey Jack cheese, and remaining ¼ cup cilantro; set aside.
4. Coat a 9x13 inch casserole dish with non-stick cooking spray. Arrange 3 of the cooked lasagna noodles in the bottom of the dish, cutting to fit if necessary. Spread with ⅓ of the bean mixture, then ⅓ of the cheese mixture. Repeat layers twice more.
5. Cover and bake in preheated oven for 45 minutes. Garnish with sliced black olives and sprigs of parsley.

Crohn's Disease and IBS: Not recommended.
Sugar 5 gms; **Fat** 6 gms

Diabetes: Replace the lasagna noodles with rice noodles. Avoid the olives.
Carbs 21 gms; **Calories** 126

Heart Disease: Avoid the olives.
Sodium 54 mgs; **Cholesterol** 15 mgs

PIZZA (for two 12-inch round pies)

Healthier pizza should have a thin crust, small amount of low-fat cheese, lots of tomato or sauce, and toppings of only vegetables, ground turkey, or chicken.

Dough:
1 cup warm (not cold) water
1 package active dry yeast
1 teaspoon sugar or baking Splenda
1 teaspoon salt
2 tablespoons extra virgin olive oil
2 cups all-purpose, unbleached flour (organic)
Additional 1½ cups all-purpose, unbleached flour (organic)

Temp: 400°
Time: 25 minutes
Yields: 16 slices

Directions:
1. Sprinkle yeast into cup of warm water.
2. Stir in sugar, salt, and oil.
3. Add 2 cups flour, beat until smooth.
4. Gradually add the additional 1½ cups flour.
5. Dough should be as soft as biscuit dough.
6. Turn out on lightly floured board and knead until smooth and elastic.
7. Place in greased bowl; brush top with shortening.
8. Cover and let rise in warm place (85 degrees) for 45 minutes.
9. Divide dough; place on greased baking sheet.
10. Press out into circles about 12-inch in diameter, making edge thin.

Topping:
1 (6-ounce) can tomato paste
½ cup water
1 teaspoon salt
Dash of pepper
1 teaspoon crushed oregano
¼ pound low-fat grated mozzarella cheese
2 tablespoons salad oil
1 (4 ounce) can mushrooms, stems and pieces (inexpensive when you buy stems and pieces, packed in water) and vegetables such as broccoli, onions, mushrooms
4 tablespoons grated reduced-fat Parmesan cheese
Green pepper, optional
Cubes of leftover meat (chicken or turkey)

continued on next page

Sauce Directions:
1. Mix together tomato paste, ½ cup water, salt, oregano, and pepper.
2. On each circle of dough, arrange half tomato paste mixture.
3. Add vegetables and meat you want to use as toppings (broccoli, onions, turkey, etc).
4. Sprinkle with Parmesan cheese and salad oil or olive oil.
5. On each circle of dough arrange half of the mozzarella cheese.
6. Bake.

Crohn's Disease and IBS:
Only use nondairy cheese.
Sugar 1 gm; **Fat** 7 gms

Diabetes:
Use baking Splenda.
Carbs 14 gms; **Calories** 59

Heart Disease:
Eliminate the salt. Use low-fat, low-sodium cheese.
Sodium 37 mgs; **Cholesterol** 5 mgs

EGGS

Eggs have a very high quality protein and can be used in the place of meat. One egg is equal to one ounce of meat, poultry or fish. They are the least expensive of all the protein foods and there is no waste. Eggs contain all nutrients except vitamin C.

While in high school my sister, Jacqui and I used to grade eggs for a neighbor. We had to pass each egg over a light (candling) to see how big the air sack was to determine the egg's freshness. Then the egg would go along a conveyer belt and drop into slots according to its weight.

Eggs are graded according to their weight, not their size:

Jumbo (30 ounces)	Medium (21 ounces)
X-Large (27 ounces)	Small (18 ounces)
Large (24 ounces)*	Pee wee (15 ounces)

* The large egg is the standard weight used in most recipes.

The cholesterol of the egg (213mg) is found in the yolk. The majority of the vitamins and minerals and 44% of the protein are also found in the yolk. There is no cholesterol in the white of the egg. It does contain protein, minerals, niacin and riboflavin. In one large egg there are 17 calories in the egg white and 59 calories in the egg yolk.

BUYING EGGS

When buying eggs, make sure the outside shell is not shiny. Shininess indicates that the egg has been washed, thus removing the outside protective coating. This will allow bacteria to enter through the pores. Check to make sure there are no cracked or broken eggs. Always buy eggs that are stored in the refrigerator case. Check the expiration date on the carton.

Eggs are AA, A (eggs that hold their shape) or B (softer, more fragile shells).

STORING EGGS

Always store eggs in the original carton with the small point of the egg facing down. They will last for 3 weeks in the refrigerator. Never leave hard cooked eggs out of the refrigerator for more than 2 hours. Refrigerate any foods containing eggs immediately. To store leftover egg yolks, cover with a small amount of water and store in a tightly sealed container in the refrigerator.

Eggs may be frozen as follows:

1. Gently break the yolk and mix with the white (Don't whip. You don't want air in them.)
2. Sprinkle with a pinch of salt.
3. Pour into plastic ice cube trays…add a little water.
4. Freeze.
5. When frozen, pop eggs out of trays and store in freezer bags.
6. They will keep for 6 months.
7. To thaw, place eggs in a dish in the refrigerator. Use immediately.
8. In a recipe, 2 cubes measures the same as 1 large egg.

COOKING

Eggs are high in protein and should be cooked on medium or low heat, but cooked thoroughly. Contrary to what many people believe, you never boil a hard or soft cooked egg.

COMPOSITION OF AN EGG

Shell: The shell is the outside covering of the egg. One of the most asked questions about eggs is, why are some eggs brown and some eggs white? It's the breed of the hen that determines the color of the eggs. Hens with red feathers and red ear lobes lay brown eggs. Hens with white feathers and white ear lobes lay white eggs. There is no difference in the nutritive value. Brown hens are larger than their white relatives and require more food. For that reason, brown eggs are more expensive than white eggs. By the way, have you ever seen a blue-green egg? The Araucana hen from South America lays blue-green eggs. They have been bred in the United States since the 30's. They are called the Ameraucanas. These chickens have no tails and have tufts of feathers that grow straight out of their ear lobes. These chickens have been referred to as the Easter egg chicken.

Yolk: The yellow of the egg is in the yolk. That's where you will find the cholesterol. One large egg contains 213 mg cholesterol. The color of the yolk is determined by the feed of the hens. Have you ever hard cooked an egg and found a greenish ring around the yolk? When eggs are overcooked, or you have a high iron count in your cooking water, iron and sulfur in the egg reacts with the surface of the yolk and turns it greenish. To avoid this, use proper termperature and cooking time. Also cool rapidly.

Vitelline (yolk membrane): A clear seal that holds the egg yolk.

Chalaza: The twisted cordlike strand that holds the egg yolk in the center of the egg. No, it isn't the beginning of an embryo.

Air Cell: The air cell is located at the large end of the egg. The small point should be facing down. As the egg gets older, the air cell gets bigger.

Shell Membrane: This membrane provides a barrier against bacteria. There is an inner and outer shell membrane surrounding the egg white.

Thin Albumen (white): This white is nearest to the shell.

Thick Albumen (white): This is the major source of protein. The white stands higher in higher grade eggs.

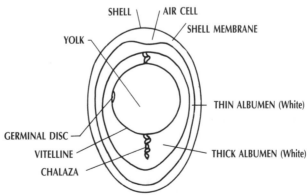

HARD COOKED EGG

Ingredients:
1 egg
Water

Temp: Medium to high
Time: 15-20 minutes
Yields: 1 serving

Directions:
1. Place eggs in saucepan and cover completely with cold water (to prevent cracking).
2. Bring eggs to the boiling point. DO NOT BOIL!
3. Take pan off the heat and let stand covered for 15-20 minutes.
4. Immediately place eggs under cold water to stop cooking action. This will keep your yolk from turning dark. The egg will also be easier to shell.
5. If you boil an egg, you destroy the protein and toughen the whites.

Crohn's Disease and IBS:
Eat only the egg whites.
Sugar 0 gms; **Fat** 5 gms

Diabetes:
Enjoy!
Carbs 0 gms; **Calories** 78

Heart Disease:
Use only the cooked white of the egg.
Sodium 55 mgs; **Cholesterol** 0 mgs

SOFT COOKED EGG

Ingredients:
1 egg
Water

Temp: Medium
Time: 2-4 minutes
Yields: 1 serving

Directions:
1. Place egg in a saucepan and cover completely with cold water.
2. Bring water just to boiling point. DO NOT BOIL!
3. Take pan off the heat and cover and let it stand for 2-4 minutes.
4. Immediately rinse under cold water to prevent eggs from over cooking.
5. Crack shell, scoop out, and serve.

Crohn's Disease and IBS:
Eat only the egg whites.
Sugar 0 gms; **Fat** 5 gms

Diabetes:
Limit intake of whole eggs.
Carbs 0 gms; **Calories** 78

Heart Disease:
Eat only the egg whites.
Sodium 55 mgs; **Cholesterol** 0 mgs

SHIRRED EGGS

Ingredients:
1 egg
1 slice of whole grain bread
1 teaspoon Smart Balance trans fat-free margarine or butter
1 teaspoon low-fat milk
Salt and pepper to taste

Temp: 350°
Time: 15 to 20 minutes
Yields: 1 serving

Directions:
1. Cut the crust off a slice of bread and butter it with trans fat-free margarine or butter. Place the buttered side down in a custard cup or muffin pan.
2. Break an egg and drop into the center of the bread.
3. Sprinkle with a pinch of salt and pepper.
4. Bake at 350° for 15-20 minutes.

Crohn's Disease and IBS:
Eat only the egg whites. Use nondairy milk.
Sugar 0 gms; **Fat** 5 gms

Diabetes:
Use a gluten-free bread and eliminate the salt and use skim milk.
Carbs 10 gms; **Calories** 71

Heart Disease:
Only use egg whites or egg substitute. Use low-sodium bread and skim milk.
Sodium 58 mgs; **Cholesterol** 0 mgs

EGG IN A FRAME

Ingredients:
Slice of whole grain bread per person
1 teaspoon trans fat-free margarine or butter
1 egg
Pinch salt and pepper

Temp: Medium to low
Time: 3-5 minutes
Yields: 1 serving

Directions:
1. Cut a shape out of the bread using a 3-inch cookie cutter.
2. Place the teaspoon of butter or margarine in the bottom of a frying pan, medium to low heat.
3. Break an egg into the center of the cut out shape.
4. Sprinkle the egg with salt and pepper.
5. Cook until the bread is toasted and the bottom of the egg is cooked.
6. Flip the toast and egg and cook over low heat for a minute.
7. Serve.

Crohn's Disease and IBS:
Use an egg substitute in the center of the bread.
Sugar 0 gms; **Fat** 5 gms

Diabetes:
Use the egg substitute in the center of the gluten-free bread.
Carbs 0 gms; **Calories** 27

Heart Disease:
Eliminate the salt and use egg substitute in the center of the bread. Use low-sodium bread.
Sodium 100 mgs; **Cholesterol** 0 mgs

OMELET

Ingredients:
2 eggs
1 tablespoon water
Pinch of salt and pepper
1 teaspoon butter or trans fat-free margarine per omelet
Desired fillings…veggies, fruits, etc.

Temp: Med to low
Time: 10 minutes
Yields: 1 serving

Directions:
1. In a small bowl, mix the eggs, water, salt, and pepper.
2. In a small, non-stick frying pan, melt the butter or margarine.
3. Pour the egg mixture into the pan so it coats the bottom.
4. Move the pan in a circular motion.
5. Using the back end of a spatula, push the cooked egg to the center and let the uncooked egg flow onto the pan.
6. Place the desired filling onto one side of the omelet and let it cook for another 2 minutes.
7. Flip the omelet in half.
8. Serve.

Crohn's Disease and IBS:
Replace the eggs with an egg substitute or egg white.
Sugar 0 gms; **Fat** 7 gms

Diabetes:
Replace the eggs with egg substitute or all egg whites. Use Smart Balance margarine and low-carb bread.
Carbs 5 gms; **Calories** 34

Heart Disease:
Replace the eggs with egg substitute or egg whites. Use a heart-safe margarine (Promise) and low-sodium bread.
Sodium 100 mgs; **Cholesterol** 0 mgs

NUTS – FAT & CALORIES

Nuts contain mostly monounsaturated fat, which doesn't raise blood cholesterol levels. Nuts are a good source of protein and vitamin E, which some studies suggest may improve the immune system.

Nuts contain at least 70% of their calories from fat, so go lightly on the amount consumed.

Listed are estimates of regular roasted nuts. Note the label as the amount may vary according to preparation. For example, some nuts are dry roasted, which significantly can lower fat and calories. Some nuts are coated with special spices and seasonings, which can increase calories and fat. Again, read the label for specific calorie and fat grams per ounce.

Nuts (1 ounce or about ¼ cup)	**Calories**	**Fat Grams**
Almonds	165	15
Brazil nuts	185	19
Cashews	165	13
Filberts (hazelnuts)	180	18
Macadamia nuts	205	22
Peanuts	165	14
Pine nuts	160	17
Pistachios	165	17
Walnuts, black	170	16
Walnuts, English	180	18

Eat a hand full of almonds or walnuts each day.

BEEF, POULTRY, AND SEAFOOD STOCKS

Soup stocks are readily available in your favorite grocery stores. I have found that making my own is not only tastier, but also more economical and nutritious. I make stock and save it in the freezer. These are the ingredients in a well-known chicken broth from the grocery store: chicken broth, contains less than 1% of the following ingredients: salt, dextrose, monosodium glutamate, hydrolyzed wheat gluten, natural flavor, water, onion juice concentrate, carrot and carrot juice concentrate, mono and diglycerides, partially hydrogenated soybean oil. A ready-made chicken bouillon cube includes the following: natural flavor, salt, sugar, chicken fat, onion, maltodextrin, chicken broth, spice, garlic, parsley, disodium guanylate (flavor enhancers). When you make your own stock you know what is in it. My mom always said, "if you can't pronounce what is in the ingredients, don't eat it." Making your own stock is not difficult and you use up leftovers that you would have otherwise thrown away.

If you want to intensify the flavor of any of your stocks just cook them down to reduce the liquid.

Soups and stews should never boil, just simmer.

If you have too much salt in your stock or soup, add a slice of raw potato, it will absorb the salt.

BEEF STOCK

Ingredients:

2 quarts of water

Leftover roast beef, beef bones, doggie bags of meat when you go out to eat (cut into cubes). A pound of beef and bones will yield a quart of stock.

2 stalks of celery

2 or 3 carrots

2 onions

Some parsley

2 cloves garlic

pepper to taste

Use any leftover veggies

Temp: Medium
Time: 1 hour
Yields: 8 servings

Directions:

1. Use a large stock pot.
2. To get a richer color, cut up the meat, flour it and brown it in a little cooking spray. Let it stick onto the bottom of the pan and deglaze it with a little water. Then add the 2 quarts of water.
3. Add all the other ingredients and simmer for 1 hour.
4. Strain out all the non-liquid ingredients.
5. Cool to get rid of any fat. Skim it off the top of the stock.
6. Use this clear stock for soups and stews. Store in freezer.
7. If desired, salt may be added when used in soups, etc.

Chill and skim off fats in soups and stews.

POULTRY STOCK

Ingredients:
3 pounds of poultry cut up or the leftover turkey or chicken carcass
3 quarts cold water
2 stalks of celery
5 carrots
2 onions
Pepper
Leftover veggies

Temp: Medium
Time: 1 hour
Yields: 6-8 servings

Directions:
1. Combine all the ingredients in a stockpot.
2. Simmer for 1 hour.
3. Skim the froth and throw away.
4. Strain out all the nonliquid ingredients.
5. Refrigerate to congeal the fat, and discard before you use the stock.
6. Freeze for use in stocks and stews.
7. If desired, salt may be added when used in soups, etc.

Vitamin B is water-soluble, so all the vitamins in the vegetables go into the stock.

SEAFOOD STOCK

Ingredients:
4 pounds mild white fish (haddock, flounder, sole, etc.)
Cooking spray
2 large onions, chopped
4 cloves garlic
1 stalk celery
Parsley
1 tablespoon lemon juice
Pepper to taste
1 gallon water

Temp: Medium to low
Time: ½ hour
Yields: 6 servings

Directions:
1. Spray stockpot.
2. Sauté onions and celery.
3. Add remaining ingredients.
4. Simmer for 1 hour.
5. Cool and strain out solid ingredients.
6. Freeze for use in soups and stews.
7. If desired, salt may be added when used in soups, etc.

VEGETABLE SOUP

Delicious and nutritious.

Ingredients:
2 tablespoons extra virgin olive oil
1 large clove garlic, minced
$\frac{1}{2}$ cup onions, chopped
2 leeks (white part, chopped)
2 carrots, diced
2 potatoes, diced
2 stalks celery, diced
$\frac{1}{4}$ cup diced eggplant
2 tomatoes, peeled and chopped (can use small can of tomatoes)
$\frac{1}{2}$ cup diced zucchini
2 pieces sweet basil
2 cups of chicken broth or stock (that you made and froze)
$\frac{1}{2}$ cup small pasta
$1\frac{1}{2}$-2 cups cooked, diced chicken
Salt and pepper to taste

Temp: Medium heat
Time: 25 minutes
Yields: 8 servings or more

Directions:
1. In a large cooking pot, place the olive oil and sauté onions, celery, garlic, leeks, and carrots until tender.
2. Add the remaining diced vegetables.
3. Add the water and chicken stock.
4. Cook for 25 minutes or until all the vegetables are tender.
5. Add the pasta.
6. Simmer until the pasta is cooked.
7. Add the cooked diced chicken.
8. Season with salt and pepper to taste.

Crohn's Disease and IBS: Cook the leeks, celery, and onions separately in water. Discard vegetables. Add water to soup pot.
Sugar 2 gms; **Fat** 8 gms

Diabetes: Use soy or rice pasta.
Carbs 14 gms; **Calories** 40

Heart Disease: Eliminate the salt.
Sodium 21 mgs; **Cholesterol** 15 mgs

BROCCOLI AND CHEESE SOUP

This recipe comes from Capriland's Herb Farm in Coventry, CT. Delicious!

Ingredients:
10 ounces fresh or frozen broccoli (finely chopped)
½ stick light butter (4 tablespoons) or Smart Balance
2 cups grated, low-fat, sharp cheese
1 (10¾-ounce) can low-sodium cream of chicken soup
½ cup leeks, chopped
½ soup can of ale
1 cup cream (half and half)
1 teaspoon paprika
2 teaspoons parsley

Temp: Medium-low heat
Time: 10 minutes
Yields: 6-8 servings

Directions:
1. Sauté broccoli in butter.
2. Add the rest of the ingredients and simmer. (Do not boil.)

Crohn's Disease and IBS:
Not recommended.
Sugar 1 gm; **Fat** 24 gms

Diabetes:
Substitute low-fat cheese for sharp cheese, low-fat cream of mushroom soup, and substitute trans fat-free margarine for butter.
Carbs 1 gm; **Calories** 88

Heart Disease:
Change butter to heart-safe margarine. The soup should be low-salt, low-fat. Substitute the low-fat cheese for the sharp cheese.
Sodium 44 mgs; **Cholesterol** 9 mgs

ITALIAN WEDDING SOUP

Ingredients:
12 ounces lean ground beef (98%, plus 2 tablespoons canola oil)
1 medium onion, chopped
2 cloves garlic, minced
4 cups beef stock (homemade from page 209)
2 cups water
1 teaspoon dried oregano, crushed
1 bay leaf (remove before serving)
½ cup cooked orzo pasta
4 cups shredded spinach
¼ teaspoon black pepper
3 ounces low-fat Parmesan cheese

Temp: Medium high
Time: 25 minutes
Yields: 8 servings

Directions:
1. Cook meat, onions, and garlic in a large, uncovered saucepan for 5 minutes, stirring occasionally.
2. Add broth, water, and spices. Bring to a boil then reduce heat.
3. Cover and simmer for 10 minutes.
4. Stir in orzo and reduce heat to medium and cook uncovered about 5 minutes until pasta is heated.
5. Remove from heat and stir in spinach.
6. Cover and let spinach cook an additional 5 minutes.
7. Serve with cheese.

Crohn's Disease and IBS:
Substitute a nondairy cheese for the Parmesan cheese. If you have trouble with kidney stones, eliminate the spinach. It's high in oxalates.
Sugar 3 gms; **Fat** 4 gms

Diabetes:
Use rice or soy pasta.
Carbs 3 gms; **Calories** 25

Heart Disease:
Substitute low-fat cheese for Parmesan cheese. If you are on a blood thinner, avoid spinach, as it contains vitamin K (promotes blood clotting).
Sodium 38 mgs; **Cholesterol** 29 mgs

LENTIL SOUP

Ingredients:
Ham bone (leftover)
1 (7-ounce) package dried lentils
Ham scraps (leftover from ham dinner)
1 medium onion, chopped
1 carrot, chopped
Salt and pepper to taste

Temp: Medium to low
Time: 2 hours, 20 minutes
Yields: 6 servings

Directions:
1. Cook ham bone in water (enough to cover bone) for 1½ hours.
2. Strain stock; chill overnight.
3. Soak lentils overnight.
4. Skin fat from stock.
5. Cook lentils in stock for 2 hours over low heat.
6. Add ham, vegetables, and seasonings.
7. Cook for 20 minutes, or until vegetables are tender.
8. Serve hot.

Crohn's Disease and IBS:
Not recommended.
Sugar 1 gm; **Fat** 2 gms

Diabetes:
Use low-salt, low-fat ham.
Carbs 3 gms; **Calories** 43

Heart Disease:
Eliminate the salt and use a low-salt, low-fat ham.
Sodium 11 mgs; **Cholesterol** 7 mgs

CHICKEN SOUP

Ingredients:

1 onion chopped
1 full stalk celery, diced
1 small clove garlic, minced
Cooking spray
4 cups homemade chicken stock (see page 210)
2 cups water
2 large carrots, diced
2 small potatoes, diced
Salt and pepper to taste
$\frac{1}{2}$ teaspoon thyme
$\frac{1}{2}$ teaspoon parsley
2 cups cut up cooked chicken
1 cup cooked no-yolk noodles

Temp: Medium
Time: $\frac{1}{2}$ hour
Yields: 6 servings

Directions:

1. Spray large saucepan with cooking spray. Sauté onions, celery and garlic.
2. Add chicken stock and water to saucepan.
3. Add carrots and potatoes to stock. Cook until vegetables are tender.
4. Sprinkle in the salt, pepper, thyme and parsley. Taste, and add more if needed.
5. Five minutes before serving add noodles and chicken.
6. Serve hot.

Crohn's Disease and IBS:
Peel and chop celery very fine.
Sugar 3 gms; **Fat** 3 gms

Diabetes:
Substitute rice or soy pasta for the no-yolk noodles.
Carbs 11 gms; **Calories** 101

Heart Disease:
Eliminate the salt. Let the soup stay in the refrigerator overnight so the fat will harden and be removed.
Sodium 24 mgs; **Cholesterol** 9 mgs

VEGETABLE BEEF SOUP

Ingredients:
3 pounds beef shank with marrow
2 quarts cold water
$^1/_2$ cup celery tops, chopped
$^1/_2$ cup celery stalks, chopped
1 medium onion, chopped
1 cup carrots, sliced
$^1/_2$ cup drained, chopped tomatoes
$^1/_2$ cup leftover vegetables
$^1/_2$ cup raw brown rice
Salt and pepper to taste

Temp: Medium to low
Time: $1^1/_2$ to 2 hours
Yields: 8 servings

Directions:
1. Bring to a boil the water, beef, celery, onion, salt, and pepper.
2. Cut beef into bite size pieces.
3. Simmer slowly for 2 hours.
4. Add the carrots, tomatoes, leftover vegetables, and rice.
5. Simmer until vegetables are tender and rice is cooked (about 35 minutes).

Crohn's Disease and IBS:
Use celery powder.
Sugar 1 gm; **Fat** 4 gms

Diabetes:
Enjoy!
Carbs 5 gms; **Calories** 48

Heart Disease:
Eliminate the salt.
Sodium 19 mgs; **Cholesterol** 6 mgs

POTATO SOUP

Ingredients:
1 onion
1 tablespoon extra virgin olive oil
4 medium potatoes
1 cup water
2 cups low-fat milk
1 teaspoon salt
Pepper to taste

Temp: Medium to low
Time: 15 to 20 minutes
Yields: 4 servings

Directions:
1. Chop onions and cook, in olive oil, until tender.
2. Cut potatoes into small pieces and add to onions.
3. Add water, cover, and boil gently for 15 minutes.
4. Mash potato mixture with fork without draining.
5. Add milk, salt, pepper and stir while heating.
6. Serve hot.

Crohn's Disease and IBS:
Use a nondairy milk.
Sugar 2 gms; **Fat** 5 gms

Diabetes:
Use a low-fat or skim milk.
Carbs 16 gms; **Calories** 135

Heart Disease:
Use skim milk, and use a favorite spice instead of salt.
Sodium 50 mgs; **Cholesterol** 2 mgs

CANADIAN PEA SOUP

Ingredients:
2 cups dried green peas
3 quarts cold water
2 small ham hocks or leftover ham bone
1 onion, chopped
1 tablespoon butter or trans fat-free margarine
1 tablespoon all-purpose, unbleached flour (organic)
1 small carrot (optional)
Salt and pepper to taste

Temp: Medium heat
Time: Simmer 4 hours
Yields: 8+ servings

Directions:
1. Soak peas in 3 quarts of water overnight.
2. Drain peas in the morning.
3. Put peas in a large pot with 2 quarts of water.
4. Add the carrot, onions, and ham hocks or ham bone.
5. Simmer about 4 hours.
6. Remove ham hock and shred meat, return meat to pot.
7. Sprinkle with salt and pepper.
8. Melt butter, stir in flour, mix until smooth.
9. Add above mixture to thicken soup, stirring constantly.
10. Serve with cornbread. (see recipe on page 90)

Crohn's Disease and IBS:
Not recommended.
Sugar 1 gm; **Fat** 3 gms

Diabetes:
Use trans fat-free margarine. Substitute rice flour for white flour.
Carbs 11 gms; **Calories** 40

Heart Disease:
Use a heart-safe margarine (Promise). Eliminate the salt in this recipe. Use a low-fat, low-salt ham.
Sodium 6 mgs; **Cholesterol** 1 mg

NEW ENGLAND CORN CHOWDER

Ingredients:
¼ cup salt pork finely chopped*
1 small onion, chopped
2 cups diced raw potatoes
1 cup water
1 can cream-styled corn (1-pound can)
1 quart low-fat milk
Salt and pepper to taste

Temp: Medium low
Time: 20 minutes
Yields: 6-8 servings

Directions:
1. Fry salt pork or bacon until brown, drain off fat by chilling.
2. Add onions and cook until tender.
3. Next add the potatoes, water, salt, and pepper.
4. Cook 15 minutes.
5. Stir in milk and corn and continue cooking until potatoes are tender.
6. Heat to serving temperature.

Canadian bacon may be used in the place of salt pork – less fat.

Crohn's Disease and IBS:
Not recommended.
Sugar 9 gms; **Fat** 2 gms

Diabetes:
Use low-fat or skim milk and Canadian bacon in place of salt pork. Corn is high in sugar.
Carbs 18 gms; **Calories** 68

Heart Disease:
Eliminate the salt pork and salt. Use a low-sodium corn.
Sodium 17 mgs; **Cholesterol** 4 mgs

FISH CHOWDER

Ingredients:

2 tablespoons chopped salt pork or Canadian bacon
2 pounds cleaned fish (Haddock or Cod)
2 small onions
4 cups potatoes
1½ cups water
Salt and pepper to taste
2½ cups low-fat milk

Temp: Medium and low heat
Time: 15 to 20 minutes
Yields: 6 to 8 servings

Directions:

1. Cut fish into small pieces.
2. Chop onions and potatoes.
3. Sauté salt pork or Canadian bacon over medium heat until brown.
4. Add onions and cook until tender.
5. Combine water, potatoes, fish, and seasonings.
6. Cover and cook over low heat until the potatoes are tender – 15 minutes, then stir in milk.
7. Serve hot.

Crohn's Disease and IBS:
Use nondairy milk. Use Canadian bacon in place of salt pork.
Sugar 5 gms; **Fat** 2 gms

Diabetes:
Use low-fat or skim milk. Use Canadian bacon in place of salt pork.
Carbs 12 gms; **Calories** 82

Heart Disease:
Eliminate the salt pork and salt. Use Canadian bacon.
Sodium 46 mgs; **Cholesterol** 3 mgs

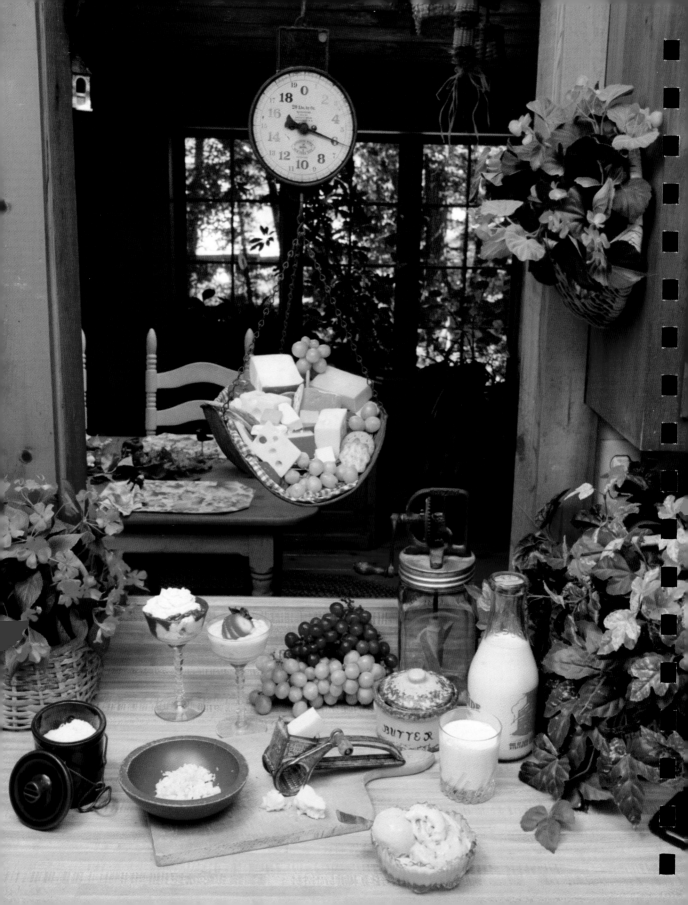

Chapter 5
MILK, YOGURT AND CHEESE GROUP

Why eat foods from the milk group?

Foods from this food group provide us with vitamin D and calcium essential for strong bones and teeth. Vitamin D regulates the utilization of calcium. Milk is one of the richest sources of calcium. Buying milk today isn't as simple as it was in the good old days, when the milkman would deliver whole milk and cream to your house. Today we have a wide variety of milk available at grocery stores. In addition to whole milk (high in fat), we have many other choices such as, reduced-fat (2%), low-fat (1%), nonfat skim milk, organic, lactose-free milk, powdered nonfat dry milk, evaporated and condensed milk. Organic milk comes from cows whose feed is free from fertilizers and pesticides. They are also not injected with hormones.

Contrary to what most people think, buttermilk is low-fat or skim milk to which a lactic acid culture is added.

Evaporated milk is milk with approximately half its water removed. It is canned and heat sterilized. Evaporated milk may be stored at room temperature.

Sweetened condensed milk is made the same way as evaporated, except sugar is added, making it high in calories.

While growing up in Maine, I lived in the country on a farm. We had an empty barn we wanted to fill with animals. Little by little we added chickens, a pig, and rabbits. We were always bringing stray animals home. One of our neighbors had a granddaughter visiting for the summer. Mary couldn't drink cow's milk and only drank goat's milk as it was easier for her to digest. Grandpa went out and bought a goat for her. When Mary went back to California at the end of the summer, Grandpa asked my sister and me if we wanted "Nanny". Well what do you think we said? We knew if mom and dad let us keep it overnight, it was ours. The condition was that we would have to feed and milk "Nanny" every day. By the way, goats don't eat tin cans! Goat's milk is slightly higher in calcium and contains about the same amount of lactose as cow's milk. Studies have not proven that goat's milk is better for lactose-intolerant people. If you drink goat's milk, make sure it's pasteurized, as it could contain bacteria.

When choosing cheese, make sure it's low-fat or fat-free. The protein in cheese puts it in the class with meat, poultry, eggs, and fish. As a milk based product, cheese is a concentrated source of all the nutrients found in milk. Cheese bought in blocks is cheaper than sliced cheese.

Grocery stores also carry nondairy drinks, such as fortified soy, rice, and almond milks. They have a similar flavor and consistency and can be used the same way as milk, for those with lactose intolerance.

Yogurt has become very popular as a diet food. There are two different styles, 1) stir, and 2) set. It's available in various flavors. Yogurt is a fermented dairy product made by adding a good bacteria culture to milk. It transforms the milk sugar into lactic acid. Yogurt is a good source of calcium, vitamins B, B_5, B_{12}, zinc, potassium, and good natural bacteria. Yogurt is believed to help the immune system.

STORAGE

Fresh milk should be stored in the refrigerator as soon as possible. Nutrients in milk are destroyed by heat and light. Milk will absorb odors, so make sure it is tightly sealed. Milk may be frozen (allow room for it to expand) but it may not taste the same. Use in cooking. Pasteurized milk can be stored in the freezer six to eight months.

Yogurt, sour cream, and cottage cheese will stay fresher if stored upside down.

Cheese should also be tightly covered and stored in the refrigerator. Freezing damages the texture of most cheeses. There are some exceptions... grated mozzarella can be frozen. Provolone, Swiss and cheddar are some of the others that may be frozen if cut in small pieces or grated. Wrap tightly in freezer paper and freeze at 0°F or lower. Use immediately when thawed.

Cheese is an excellent food by itself and is also an ingredient in many recipes. When cheese is served as an appetizer it should be at room temperature for the fullest flavor. The only exceptions are cream cheese and cottage cheese, which should be refrigerated until serving to prevent spoilage.

COOKING

Use nonfat dry milk fortified with vitamin A and D. It costs less than whole milk and you cannot taste the difference.

When scalding milk, add a teaspoon of water to prevent a skin from forming.

DRINKING

Mix $\frac{1}{2}$ whole milk with $\frac{1}{2}$ nonfat milk and make sure it is well chilled.

HINTS

One quart of evaporated milk is equal to three quarts of whole milk, and is approximately $\frac{1}{2}$ the cost.

224

BLUEBERRY COOLER

Ingredients: **Yields:** 4 servings

6 ounces blueberry fat-free yogurt
1 cup fresh or frozen blueberries
1 cup orange juice
2 scoops lemon sherbet

Directions:
1. Mix the yogurt, blueberries, and juice in a blender.
2. Add the lemon sherbet and blend.
3. Pour into glasses.
4. Serve cooled.

Crohn's Disease and IBS:
Substitute sorbet for sherbet.
Sugar 15 gms; **Fat** 1 gms

Diabetes:
Ok to drink.
Carbs 32 gms; **Calories** 79

Heart Disease:
Ok to drink.
Sodium 29 mgs; **Cholesterol** 0 mgs

SUMMER SHAKE

Ingredients:
6 ounce nonfat strawberry or vanilla yogurt
1 cup fruit in season (strawberries, raspberries, etc.)
½ banana
Granola (see recipe on page 101)

Yields: 2 servings (8 ounces)

Directions:
1. Place yogurt into blender.
2. Add fruit and ½ banana.
3. Blend together.
4. Place in 2 glasses.
5. Sprinkle the granola on top.
6. Serve cooled.

Crohn's Disease and IBS:
Eliminate the granola. Use tofu ice cream.
Sugar 14 gms; **Fat** 2 gms

Diabetes:
Eliminate the granola.
Carbs 26 gms; **Calories** 148

Heart Disease:
Enjoy.
Sodium 42 mgs; **Cholesterol** 2 mgs

Strawberry

4 cups low-fat or no fat milk
Large scoop low-fat frozen strawberry yogurt
$1/2$ teaspoon pure vanilla extract
1 teaspoon sugar
1 cup frozen or fresh strawberries

Chocolate

$3/4$ cup 1% milk
1 pint frozen chocolate yogurt
3 tablespoons chocolate syrup

Vanilla

4 cups low-fat milk
Large scoop vanilla yogurt
1 teaspoon pure vanilla extract
1 teaspoon sugar or Splenda

Strawberry-Banana

2 bananas
1 cup strawberries
2 cups orange juice
$1/2$ teaspoon pure vanilla extract
Crushed ice

Peachy-Keen Cooler

1 large can peaches and its juice
2 cups frozen vanilla yogurt
4 cups nonfat milk

Purple Cow

4 cups nonfat milk
2 cups vanilla frozen yogurt
1 large can frozen grape juice

The above drinks are made in a blender. By substituting low-fat frozen yogurt in the place of ice cream, there are 0 grams of fat. In one cup of yogurt there are 452 milligrams of calcium and only 127 calories compared to 24 grams of fat, 152 milligrams of calcium, and 350 calories in regular ice cream.

Above drinks should be served cooled.

APRICOT GINGER FIZZ

Yields: 2 servings (8 ounces)

Ingredients:
6 ounces low-fat apricot yogurt
1 tablespoon lime juice
1 frozen banana
1 cup ginger ale

Directions:
1. Mix yogurt, lime juice, and banana in a blender.
2. Add a cup of ginger ale and blend.
3. Pour into glasses and serve.

Crohn's Disease and IBS:
If your Crohn's disease is active, don't drink this recipe.
Sugar 14 gms; **Fat** 0 gms

Diabetes:
Use diet ginger ale.
Carbs 12 gms; **Calories** 90

Heart Disease:
Use diet ginger ale.
Sodium 20 mgs; **Cholesterol** 0 mgs

MEXICAN CHOCOLATE DRINK

This was a favorite of my students.

Ingredients:
4 cups low-fat milk
2 ounces of milk chocolate
½ teaspoon ground cinnamon
½ teaspoon pure vanilla extract

Temp: Medium heat (8 ounces)
Yields: 4 servings

Directions:
1. Pour milk into the saucepan.
2. Add the chocolate and stir over medium heat.
3. Once the chocolate is melted, remove from heat.
4. Add the cinnamon and vanilla.
5. Serve hot.

Crohn's Disease and IBS:
Use a nondairy milk.
Sugar 2 gms; **Fat** 3 gms

Diabetes:
Replace milk with low-fat skim milk.
Carbs 21 gms; **Calories** 146

Heart Disease:
Replace milk with low-fat skim milk.
Sodium 37 mgs; **Cholesterol** 5 mgs

HOT CRAB DIP

Ingredients:

1 pound crabmeat
1 tablespoon lemon juice
6 ounces whipped low-fat cream cheese
3 tablespoons low-fat mayonnaise made with canola oil

Temp: 350°
Time: 30 minutes
Yields: 6 servings

Directions:

1. Add all the ingredients to the whipped cream cheese.
2. Bake in a small casserole dish for 30 minutes.

Crohn's Disease and IBS:
Replace cream cheese with soy cream cheese.
Sugar 0 gms; **Fat** 2 gms

Diabetes:
Enjoy!
Carbs 1 gm; **Calories** 36

Heart Disease:
Enjoy!
Sodium 39 mgs; **Cholesterol** 34 mgs

NEW ENGLAND CLAM DIP

Ingredients:
1 cup low-fat cream-style cottage cheese
1 (4-ounce) package low-fat cream cheese
2 teaspoons horseradish
1 teaspoon low-sodium Worcestershire sauce
1 cup minced clams, drained
Paprika
3 tablespoons half and half milk or low-fat milk

Temp: 350°
Time: 30 minutes
Yields: 6-8 servings

Directions:
1. Blend the cottage cheese, cream cheese, horseradish, and Worcestershire in a medium bowl.
2. Stir in the clams.
3. Chill.
4. Beat in the half and half milk.
5. Sprinkle top with paprika.

Crohn's Disease and IBS:
Not recommended.
Sugar 2 gms; **Fat** 1 gm

Diabetes:
Use all low-fat dairy products.
Carbs 1 gm; **Calories** 52

Heart Disease:
There are 65 mg of sodium in a teaspoon of Worcestershire sauce. Eliminate.
Sodium 74 mgs; **Cholesterol** 7 mgs

DILL WEED DIP

Ingredients: **Yields:** 2³/₄ cups
¹/₄ cup dill weed
1 pound soft tofu, drained
1 (8-ounce) cup plain nonfat sour cream
¹/₃ cup onion, chopped
2 tablespoons low-fat mayonnaise made with canola oil
¹/₂ teaspoon salt
Round, unsliced rye bread to be used as a container
Serve dip with vegetables

Directions:
1. In a food processor or blender, combine all ingredients until smooth.
2. Cut the top off the rye bread and remove the insides.
3. Place the dip in the hollow bread. Decorate the edge of the bread with parsley.

Crohn's Disease and IBS:
Replace sour cream with a nondairy sour cream.
Sugar 1 gm; **Fat** 5 gms

Diabetes:
Omit the salt.
Carbs 3 gms; **Calories** 36

Heart Disease:
Omit the salt. Use low-salt mayonnaise.
Sodium 7 mgs; **Cholesterol** 4 mgs

Ingredients: **Yields:** 1 cup

1 (15-ounce) can black beans, rinsed and drained
2 tablespoons onions, chopped
2 tablespoons parsley, chopped
1 tablespoon lemon juice
2 cloves minced garlic
$1/4$ teaspoon ground cumin
$1/4$ teaspoon pepper
$1/4$ cup plain nonfat yogurt
Pita crisps (recipe below)

Directions:
1. In a food processor or blender, combine the beans ,onions, parsley, lemon juice, garlic, cumin, and pepper.
2. Cover and blend until mixture is smooth.
3. Blend in the yogurt and serve with pita crisps.

PITA CRISPS

Ingredients: **Temp:** 350°
Pita rounds   **Time:** 10 minutes
                                                        Yields: 6-8 servings
Directions:
1. Cut pita bread rounds in half, horizontally; cut each half in 6-8 wedges.
2. Place pita wedge in a single layer on a ungreased baking sheet.
3. Bake uncovered until crisp.
4. Serve with the bean dip.

Crohn's Disease and IBS:
Not recommended.
Sugar 2 gms; **Fat** 2 gms

Diabetes:
Enjoy!
Carbs 5 gms; **Calories** 24

Heart Disease:
Use organic no salt added black beans. (Eden Foods)
Sodium 22 mgs; **Cholesterol** 1 mg

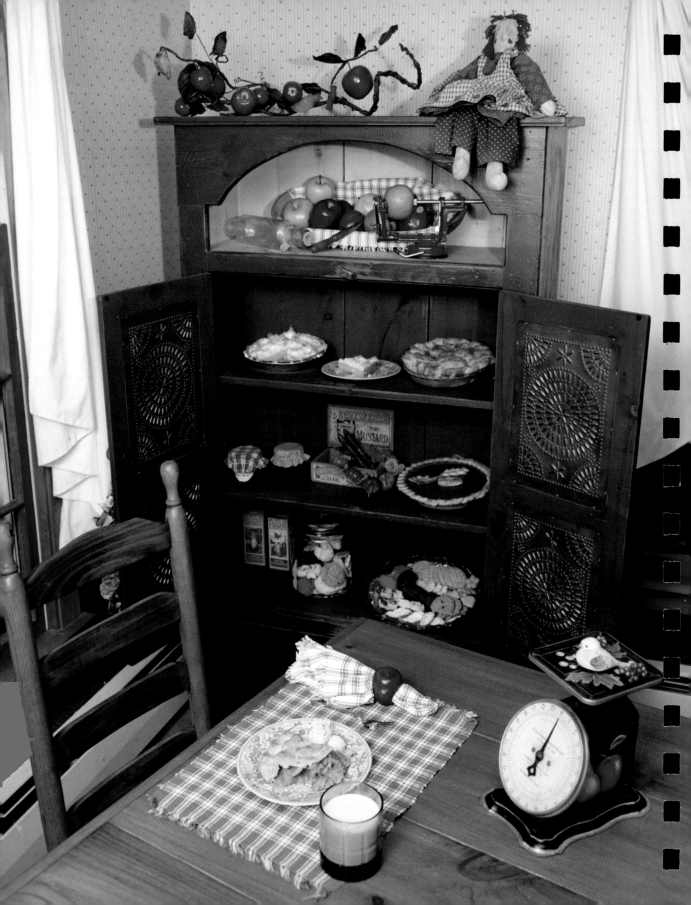

Chapter 6
FATS, OILS AND SWEETS

Why not eat foods in the fat, oil and sweets group?

Foods in this group contain empty calories. Face it, most of us enjoy the cakes, cookies, pies, puddings and candies in this group. I can say, don't eat them, but most of us will anyway. It's my goal to show you how you can eat these by making better choices. For example, if you insist on eating potato chips, at least choose the thicker ones, they absorb less grease and fat. An even better choice would be baked chips.

Limit your intake from this group and offer your children fresh cut up fruits and vegetables. They will only eat what you provide them with. If you buy them lots of sweets and fatty foods, they will be tempted to eat them.

Sugar and fat can be reduced by $\frac{1}{3}$ in most recipes. If the recipe calls for 1 cup, use only $\frac{2}{3}$ cup. Quick breads, puddings, and fruits work well with less sugar. Cookies and cakes, not as well. Applesauce may be substituted for oils in some recipes. The flavor and texture will be effected if you use less fat in some cookie and cake recipes. If everyone reduced salt, sugar, and fat from our diets, we would be so much healthier.

BUYING

Always read the label when buying any products, to see how much sugar, salt, and fat has been added. If it's the first or second ingredient, it contains too much.

Avoid ready prepared foods that contain palm oil or lard, as they are very high in saturated fats. Explain to your children why too much sugar, fat, and salt is bad for their health. Don't buy lots of candy and sweets—as they say, out of sight, out of mind. Replace some of the sugar in the recipes with vanilla and other flavorings.

There is an ongoing controversy over the health risk of artificial sweeteners. The latest is Splenda, manufactured by Johnson and Johnson. The FDA has approved it as a food. Splenda is the trade name for a new synthetic compound called sucrolose. The body does not recognize sucrolose as a food. Sucrolose contains 0 calories, 0 fat, 0 sodium, and 0 carbohydrates.

In an article written for *Women to Women*, Dr. Marcelle Pick OB/GYN NP, wrote the following: "Is Splenda safe? The truth is, we don't know yet. It's new and there are no long term studies of the side effects of Splenda in humans."

People have been using artificial sweeteners for decades. Some have been proven to be potentially unhealthy. Only long term studies will prove conclusive results to its safety. I chose to use Splenda in my recipes because it was approved by the FDA and contains 0 calories, 0 fat, 0 sodium, and 0 carbohydrates. I feel it is a better alternative to refined sugar and other artificial sweeteners.

Like any sweetener, use in moderation. Too much sugar may cause headaches, indigestion, bloating, gas and cramps.

There is a natural alternative to artificial sweeteners. It's called Stevia (sweet herb). It belongs to the Asteraceae (sunflower) family. It's a native to South and Central America. It has 0 calories and does not trigger an insulin reaction in diabetics as sugar does. It has been used in other countries for 400 years with no adverse effects. Stevia is also grown in East Asia and is popular in Japan and China.

According to Dr. Pick, "We've known about Stevia in the US since 1918, but pressure from the sugar import trade blocked its use as a commodity. Today Stevia is slowly gaining steam as a sugar substitute, despite similar hurdles. The FDA has approved its use as a food supplement, but not as a food additive due to lack of studies. Stevia can be used for anything you might use sugar in, including baking. It is naturally low in carbohydrates. You can buy Stevia at most health food stores and over the web. There will always be those who have a sensitivity to a substance, but based on reports from other countries it appears to have little to no side effects. For women who want to move through their cravings for sugar without artificial chemicals, Stevia is a great option."

Stevia may cost more than sugar, but you only need to use a small amount, as it is 20 times sweeter than sugar. One teaspoon of Stevia is equal to one cup of refined sugar. *The Stevia Cookbook*, written by Ray Sahelian and Donna Gates is available online. Other natural sweeteners are honey, molasses and maple syrup.

When using any of these recipes, choose the sweetener you feel comfortable using. Be a wise consumer and read the effects of all these sugar substitutes and natural sweeteners that you are feeding your family. Sugar comes in many forms: Dextrose, fructose (fruit) glucose, lactose (dairy products), corn syrup, honey, molasses, maple syrup, and Stevia. Some of the artificial sweeteners are: Splenda, Aspartame (NutraSweet), Cyclamates, Saccharine, and Sorbitol (can cause diarrhea). Go to the web and check out these artificial sweeteners for yourself…you will be surprised what chemicals you may be eating.

Instead of buying ready prepared desserts, make your own. You have control of what goes into your homemade products. Practice moderation when buying and eating sugar, fats, and sodium. Before using molasses or honey, spray the measuring cup with cooking spray and the molasses and honey will just slide out of the cup.

Buy oils such as canola, pure olive oil, sunflower, and safflower that are low in saturated fats. Canola oil works best, if it is to be heated at a higher temperature.

When it comes to butter or margarine I have been using a light trans fat-free margarine called Smart Balance. It's lactose-free, gluten- and dairy-free, and has 0 carbohydrates. It does contain a small amount of palm oil. Some of the other trans fat-free margarines are: Brummel and Brown Soft (made with 25% yogurt), I Can't Believe It's Not Butter Fat-Free Light, Promise (all brands), Shedd's Country Crock Squeez-able, Smart Balance (light and regular), Spectrum Spreads (all), and Olivio (made with olive oils). There are other brands of margarine and butter on the market too, choose the one you prefer.

When it comes to salt, use sparingly. Replace with spices. Do you know the difference between table salt, sea salt, and Kosher salt?

1) Table salt comes from salt mines under the ground. It has fine granules. Iodine and calcium silicate (an anti caking ingredient) are added to table salt.

2) Sea Salt is evaporated from seawater and there is little to no processing. There are no additives, and the crystals are larger.

3) Kosher Salt can come from either seawater or underground. There are no additives. It has larger irregular crystals and is excellent for curing meats.

Table salt is the least expensive of the three salts. The difference is in the taste and texture.

BUYING (continued)

All flour is not the same. To eat healthier desserts, use flour that has never been bleached or bromated. Avoid "enriched" flour. Most of the vitamins and minerals (bran and germ) have been removed. They are replaced with only a few supplements. Our bodies break down enriched flour too quickly, flooding the bloodstream with too much sugar. A healthier choice is whole grain organic flour, or all-purpose, unbleached organic flour. Arrowhead Mills spelt and whole grain organic flour may be found at health food stores.

STORAGE OF SUGAR AND OILS

Store brown sugar in a tightly covered jar. Add a slice of apple to keep the brown sugar from getting hard. The apple will also soften hard brown sugar. Store honey and molasses at room temperature.

Store oil for only a month at a time, as it can become rancid. Be sure to keep oil refrigerated once opened.

Add a few grains of rice to the salt shaker to keep salt flowing and free from condensation.

Keep whole grain flour in a tightly covered jar in the refrigerator or cool, dry, dark place.

COOKING

To reduce fat when cooking, use non-stick pans and cooking spray.

CAKE BAKING TIPS

When baking cakes, it's important to have all the ingredients at room temperature. Read the recipe, and assemble all ingredients and utensils. Be sure to preheat the oven for 10 minutes. A successful cake depends on correct blending of all the ingredients; creaming sugar with butter, as well as gently folding in egg whites to maintain maximum aeration. Measurements should be exact. Be sure to use the correct size pan called for in the recipe. Use shiny metal pans, as they will reflect the heat from the cake and cause browning. Grease the bottom and sides of the pan with shortening and dust with flour. Shake out all the excessive flour. Don't grease and dust pans when baking angel food and chiffon cakes, as they have to cling to the sides of the pan to rise properly.

Always bake cakes in the center of the oven. This will ensure good circulation of heat. A cake is done when the sides shrink back from the edge of the pan. The top should spring back when lightly pressed with the fingertips. Cool slightly before removing cake from the pan. Coat the cooling rack with cooking spray before placing the baked cake to cool.

Cool cakes thoroughly before frosting and storing, otherwise, they will become sticky.

TOMATO SOUP CAKE

Ingredients:
¹/₂ cup butter or trans fat-free margarine
³/₄ cup sugar or baking Splenda
1 can low-salt tomato soup
2 cups sifted all-purpose, unbleached flour (organic)
1 teaspoon cinnamon
1 teaspoon baking soda
2 teaspoon baking powder (aluminum-free)
1 teaspoon clove
1 teaspoon salt

Temp: 350°
Time: 35 minutes
Yields: 8 servings

Directions:
1. Cream butter and sugar until light and fluffy.
2. Combine tomato soup and creamed mixture.
3. Sift the remaining dry ingredients together.
4. Gradually add to butter mixture, beating constantly.
5. Pour into well-greased and lightly floured 10″ square cake pan.
6. Bake for 35 minutes.

Crohn's Disease and IBS:
Change the butter to trans fat-free margarine. Change sugar to baking Splenda. Ginger is good for digestion and may be substituted for the clove.
Sugar 14 gms; **Fat** 2 gms

Diabetes:
Cinnamon is good for diabetics. Substitute the sugar to baking Splenda. Replace butter with a heart-safe margarine (Promise).
Carbs 23 gms; **Calories** 189

Heart Disease:
Replace the butter with trans fat-free margarine. Use baking powder and baking soda. Eliminate salt.
Sodium 276 mgs; **Cholesterol** 0 mgs

CARROT CAKE

Ingredients:
³/₄ cup melted low-fat margarine
1 cup sugar or baking Splenda
2 eggs or 4 egg whites
1¹/₂ cups all-purpose, unbleached flour (organic)
¹/₄ teaspoon salt
1 teaspoon baking powder (aluminum-free)
¹/₄ cup grated carrots or small jar of baby food carrots
1 teaspoon cinnamon

Temp: 375°
Time: 35-45 minutes
Yields: 8 servings

Directions:
1. Blend sugar and margarine until creamed.
2. Add one egg at a time, beating well after each addition.
3. Add sifted dry ingredients and carrots alternately.
4. Place in greased 8x8 pan.
5. Bake.

Hint: Use a wet knife when cutting a cake.

Crohn's Disease and IBS:
Use the jar of baby food carrots. Use baking Splenda in place of sugar. Replace whole eggs with egg whites.
Sugar 16 gms; **Fat** 2 gms

Diabetes:
Replace sugar with baking Splenda.
Carbs 11 gms; **Calories** 65

Heart Disease:
Exchange the 2 eggs for either egg substitute or 4 egg whites. Eliminate the salt. Use heart-safe, unsalted margarine.
Sodium 2 mgs; **Cholesterol** 0 mgs

MOCK CHIFFON CAKE

Ingredients:
Beat at high speed
1 box of vanilla cake mix
2 large eggs or 4 egg whites
½ cup cooking oil
1 box instant vanilla pudding (dry)
1 teaspoon pure vanilla extract

Temp: 350°
Time: 25-35 minutes
Yields: 8 servings

Directions:
1. Mix all the above ingredients in a large mixing bowl.
2. Using an electric mixer beat ingredients at high speed.
3. Bake in a greased and floured 9x9 cake pan.
4. Do not open oven door for entire cooking time. (check through oven window)
5. Cool, then frost with cream cheese icing.

Crohn's Disease and IBS:
Not recommended.
Sugar 2 gms; **Fat** 5 gms

Diabetes:
Enjoy!
Carbs 10 gms; **Calories** 60

Heart Disease:
Replace eggs with egg substitute.
Sodium 61 mgs; **Cholesterol** 0 mgs

PENNY-WISE CAKE

Ingredients:
2 cups sifted all-purpose, unbleached flour (organic)
2 tablespoons baking powder (aluminum-free)
¼ teaspoon salt
¼ cup shortening or butter
¾ cup sugar or baking Splenda
1 egg or 2 egg whites
¾ cup low-fat milk
1 teaspoon pure vanilla extract
1 teaspoon lemon flavoring

Temp: 350°
Time: 35 minutes
Yields: 6-8 servings

Directions:
1. Sift flour with baking powder and salt.
2. Cream shortening and gradually blend in sugar.
3. Add egg and beat very thoroughly.
4. Alternately add flour mixture and milk, a small amount at a time, beating after each addition until smooth.
5. Add vanilla and lemon flavoring.
6. Pour batter into greased and floured 1½ quart ring mold.
7. Bake.

Variation: Place lemon pie filling in bottom of ring mold and let cool. Then, pour penny-wise cake filling over the filling and bake.

Crohn's Disease and IBS:
Use nondairy milk. Use egg whites in place of whole eggs. Use Splenda in place of refined sugar.
Sugar 6 gms; **Fat** 8 gms

Diabetes:
Use skim milk.
Carbs 16 gms; **Calories** 160

Heart Disease:
Replace milk with low-fat or skim milk. Use a heart-safe margarine. Eliminate the salt. Use egg whites in place of whole eggs.
Sodium 20 mgs; **Cholesterol 0 mgs**

JUDY'S CHOCOLATE QUICKIE NO-EGG CAKE

Judy and I worked our way through college, waiting on tables, during the summer. We had no money and no time. Judy's no egg cake was a wonderful low cost treat.

Ingredients:

Sift into 9" square pan:

1½ cups all-purpose, unbleached flour (organic)

½ teaspoon salt

3 tablespoons cocoa powder

½ teaspoon baking soda

1 cup sugar or baking Splenda

Make 3 holes in mixture:

In #1 hole, put 6 tablespoons cooking oil

In #2 hole, put 1 tablespoon vinegar

In #3 hole, put 1 teaspoon pure vanilla extract

Temp: 350°
Time: 35-40 minutes
Yields: 6 servings

Directions:

1. Pour 1 cup cold water over all ingredients.
2. Mix with a fork.
3. Bake.

Crohn's Disease and IBS:
Use baking Splenda in place of granular sugar.
Sugar 8 gms; **Fat** 13 gms

Diabetes:
Use the baking Splenda in place of granular sugar.
Carbs 15 gms; **Calories** 51

Heart Disease:
Eliminate the salt.
Sodium 11 mgs; **Cholesterol** 0 mgs

SIMPLE ONE EGG CAKE

Ingredients:
1¼ cups all-purpose, unbleached flour (organic)
¾ cup sugar or baking Splenda
2 teaspoons baking powder (aluminum-free)
½ teaspoon salt
⅓ cup butter, melted (or low-fat margarine)
½ cup low-fat milk
1 egg or 2 egg whites
1 teaspoon pure vanilla extract

Temp: 375°
Time: 25 minutes
Yields: 6 servings

Directions:
1. Sift dry ingredients.
2. Add melted butter, milk, egg, and vanilla.
3. Beat for 1 minute.
4. Pour into greased and floured 9″ square pan.
5. Bake.

Crohn's Disease and IBS:
Use nondairy milk substitute. Use egg whites in place of whole eggs. Replace butter with margarine.
Sugar 8 gms; **Fat** 6 gms

Diabetes:
Substitute sugar with baking Splenda.
Carbs 8 gms; **Calories** 50

Heart Disease:
Eliminate salt and use 2 egg whites in place of the whole egg. Use a heart-safe margarine.
Sodium 18 mgs; **Cholesterol** 0 mgs

OLD TIME GINGERBREAD

This recipe for gingerbread cake came over from Europe on the Mayflower, *and remains one of the favorites today.*

Ingredients:
½ cup butter or low-fat margarine
⅓ cup sugar or baking Splenda
1 egg or 2 egg whites
¾ cup molasses
1¾ cups all-purpose, unbleached flour (organic)
1 teaspoon baking powder (aluminum-free)
1 teaspoon cinnamon
1 teaspoons ginger
Pinch salt
½ cup low-fat milk

Temp: 350°
Time: 40-45 minutes
Yields: 8 servings

Directions:
1. Cream butter and sugar, add egg and molasses and mix well.
2. Sift flour, baking powder, cinnamon, ginger, and salt together.
3. Add flour mixture and milk alternately to the creamed ingredients.
4. Grease and flour an 8-inch square cake pan. Pour in gingerbread mixture.
5. Bake.

This tastes great with homemade applesauce or whipped cream.

Crohn's Disease and IBS:
Use nondairy milk and egg whites. Use baking Splenda and margarine.
Sugar 2 gms; **Fat** 8 gms

Diabetes:
Replace sugar with baking Splenda. Use skim milk and margarine.
Carbs 10 gms; **Calories** 80

Heart Disease:
Use 2 egg whites or egg substitute in place of the whole egg. Eliminate the salt, and use heart-safe margarine.
Sodium 52 mgs; **Cholesterol** 0 mgs

MELT IN YOUR MOUTH BLUEBERRY CAKE

This is a great Maine dessert made with fresh wild blueberries that are full of antioxidants. This is a very popular dessert at Maine clambakes.

Ingredients:
2 eggs or 4 egg whites
1 cup sugar or baking Splenda
¼ teaspoon salt
½ cup shortening or low-fat margarine
1 teaspoon pure vanilla extract
1½ cups all-purpose, unbleached flour (organic)
1 teaspoon baking powder (aluminum-free)
⅓ cup low-fat milk
1½ cups fresh blueberries (or frozen, not thawed)

Temp: 350°
Time: 50-60 minutes
Yields: 8 servings

Directions:
1. Beat eggs and sugar together.
2. Add margarine, salt, and vanilla to the egg mixture. Beat until creamy.
3. Add sifted dry ingredients alternately with the milk.
4. Mix blueberries in a little flour. (Flour keeps the berries evenly distributed.) Fold into batter.
5. Pour into an 8x8 lightly greased pan.
6. Sprinkle some granulated sugar over the top of the cake. (optional)
7. Bake.

Crohn's Disease and IBS:
Use nondairy milk substitute. Replace whole eggs with egg substitute. I use the small Maine wild blueberries; they are easier to digest. I buy them in the summer and freeze them for the winter months.
Sugar 6 gms; **Fat** 5 gms

Diabetes:
Replace sugar with baking Splenda. Replace milk with skim milk.
Carbs 7 gms; **Calories** 67

Heart Disease:
Replace eggs with egg substitute or 4 egg whites. Eliminate salt. Use a heart-safe margarine (Promise).
Sodium 29 mgs; **Cholesterol** 0 mgs

WILD MAINE BLUEBERRY SPICE DESSERT BREAD

This recipe is delicious! It came from the Spurwink Country Kitchen restaurant in Scarborough, Maine. It's one of their treasured family recipes.

Ingredients:
4 eggs or egg substitute
2 cups sugar or baking Splenda
1½ cups canola oil
3 cups all-purpose, unbleached flour (organic)
½ teaspoon salt
1 teaspoon baking soda
¼ teaspoon all-spice
1 teaspoon cinnamon
¼ teaspoon nutmeg
2½ cups fresh or frozen Wyman Wild Maine Blueberries

Temp: 350°
Time: 55 minutes
Yields: 2 loaves

Directions:
1. Well grease and flour 2 loaf pans.
2. Use a food processor to mix eggs, sugar and canola oil.
3. Add salt, all-spice, cinnamon and nutmeg.
4. Mix in the flour, ½ cup at a time, until well blended.
5. Add blueberries and blend until the batter turns blue.
6. Place batter into 2 well greased and floured pans.
7. Bake...DELICIOUS!

Crohn's Disease and IBS:
Eliminate the all-spice and use Splenda or Stevia in place of sugar. Use egg substitute. Blend the blueberries before adding to the batter.
Sugar 22 gms; **Fat** 0 gms

Diabetes:
Replace sugar with Spenda or Stevia. Use rice flour mixture.
Carbs 8 gms; **Calories** 34

Heart Disease:
Eliminate the salt. Replace sugar with Splenda or Stevia. Use egg substitute.
Sodium 3 mgs; **Cholesterol** 0 mgs

DOWNEAST APPLE CRISP

Ingredients:
4 cups sliced apples (Macintosh and Granny Smith)
1 teaspoon cinnamon
$^1/_2$ teaspoon salt
$^3/_4$ cup all-purpose, unbleached flour (organic)
$^1/_2$ cup sugar or Splenda
$^1/_3$ cup butter or trans fat-free margarine

Temp: 350°
Time: 35 minutes
Yields: 6 servings

Directions:
1. Preheat oven.
2. Arrange apples in the bottom of a greased 8x8x2 pan.
3. Combine the remaining ingredients with a pastry blender or fork.
4. Sprinkle mixture over the apples.
5. Bake until golden brown.
6. Serve warm with yogurt ice cream.

Crohn's Disease and IBS:
Replace sugar with Splenda or Stevia. Use a trans fat-free margarine.
Sugar 7 gms; **Fat** 1 gm

Diabetes:
Replace sugar with Splenda or Stevia. Use a trans fat-free margarine.
Carbs 9 gms; **Calories** 44

Heart Disease:
Replace sugar with Splenda or Stevia. Use a heart-safe margarine and eliminate the salt.
Sodium 35 mgs; **Cholesterol** 1 mg

SIX BASIC TYPES OF COOKIES

Bar Cookie   The bar cookie is the easiest cookie to make. It is soft dough and is spread into a baking pan. It is also the easiest to ship in the mail. A popular bar cookie is the brownie.

Drop Cookie   The drop cookie is soft dough. It should be dropped onto a shiny cookie sheet. Favorite drop cookies are chocolate chip and oatmeal raisin.

Rolled Cookie   A rolled cookie has stiff dough. It is rolled and cut into different shapes. Sugar and magic window cookies are rolled cookies.

Pressed Cookie   A pressed cookie is made with a semi-stiff dough that is put into a cookie press. These are the quickest to make and the most professional looking. Spritz cookies are the most popular pressed cookies.

Molded Cookie   A molded cookie is stiff dough that is shaped into balls and different shapes. Most peoples' favorite molded cookies are peanut butter and snicker doodles.

Refrigerator Cookies

These cookies are made with stiff dough. They are shaped into long rolls, wrapped and chilled, and put in the refrigerator. When needed, they are cut into equal slices and baked. Vanilla Crisps are a popular refrigerator cookie.

COOKIE BAKING AND STORING TIPS

Always assemble all your utensils and ingredients.

In all cookie recipes you cream shortening (margarine or butter) and sugar together.

Then add eggs and flavoring. Dry ingredients are sifted together to make sure they are well blended.

There are 2 tablespoons of extra flour in unsifted flour. If the recipe says sifted, sift before measuring. Sifting adds air to the flour and it takes less flour to fill the cup.

The dry ingredients are then added to the creamed ingredients.

Remember to only use shiny cookie sheets and do not place cold cookie dough onto a warm pan. Bake cookies on the rack in the center of the oven. There should be at least 2 inches around the cookie sheet, so the heat can circulate.

Never use a wet pot holder when you are taking a hot cookie sheet from the oven, you will get a steam burn.

Spray cooling racks with cooking spray to prevent cookies from sticking.

Completely cool cookies on a cooling rack before you store them in an airtight container. Store crisp and soft cookies in separate containers. Crisp cookies will get soft if you store them together. Soft cookies contain the most fat.

Baked cookies can be stored for a year in the freezer. Use airtight freezer containers. Your unbaked cookie dough can be stored for 6 months in the freezer.

To make your own baking Splenda, use $1/2$ Splenda and $1/2$ granulated sugar. If brown sugar or molasses are in the recipe, only replace the white sugar with Splenda.

Applesauce can be used in place of oil in some recipes. Two egg whites are the same as one whole egg in a recipe.

Never use tub margarine in recipes when baking cakes and cookies, the tubs contain too much air and water.

FUDGE BROWNIE BARS

Dark chocolate is said to contain antioxidants.

Ingredients:
½ cup butter or Smart Balance
1 cup granulated sugar or baking Splenda
2 eggs or 4 egg whites
1 teaspoon pure vanilla extract
½ cup dark cocoa powder
¼ teaspoon baking powder (aluminum-free)
½ cup sifted all-purpose, unbleached flour (organic)
½ cup chopped walnuts (optional)

Temp: 325°
Time: 30-35 minutes
Yields: 16 squares

Directions:
1. Cream butter and sugar.
2. Add eggs and vanilla.
3. Blend in the cocoa powder.
4. Add the baking powder.
5. Stir in the sifted flour.
6. Add chopped nuts.
7. Bake in a greased 8x8x2 inch square pan.
8. Cool.

Crohn's Disease and IBS:
Finely chop or eliminate the nuts. Replace eggs with 4 egg whites. Use Smart Balance and baking Splenda.
Sugar 3 gms; **Fat** 1 gm

Diabetes:
Substitute baking Splenda for white sugar.
Carbs 1 gm; **Calories** 11

Heart Disease:
Use heart-safe margarine and 4 egg whites. Use baking Splenda.
Sodium 12 mgs; **Cholesterol** 0 mgs

CAKE BROWNIES

Ingredients:
¼ cup butter or light, heart-safe margarine
1 cup granulated sugar or baking Splenda
2 egg yolks
¼ cup low-fat milk
½ teaspoon pure vanilla extract
2 (1-ounce) squares unsweetened dark chocolate, melted
⅔ cup sifted all-purpose, unbleached flour (organic)
½ teaspoon baking powder (aluminum-free)
½ teaspoon salt
⅓ cup chopped nuts (optional)
2 stiff-beaten egg whites

Temp: 350
Time: 25-30 minutes
Yields: 16 squares

Directions:
1. Cream butter and sugar until fluffy.
2. Add egg yolks, milk, and vanilla. Beat well.
3. Stir in melted chocolate.
4. Sift together dry ingredients. Add to creamed mixture and mix well.
5. Stir in chopped nuts.
6. Fold in egg whites.
7. Turn into greased and floured 9x9x2 inch baking pan.
8. Bake.

Crohn's Disease and IBS:
Use nondairy milk and finely chopped nuts. Replace squares of chocolate with unsweetened cocoa powder (3 tablespoons of cocoa and 1 tablespoon canola oil equals 1 square of chocolate). Use baking Splenda in place of sugar.
Sugar 3 gms; **Fat** 4 gms

Diabetes:
Use baking Splenda in place of white sugar. Replace skim milk for low-fat milk.
Carbs 3 gms; **Calories** 42

Heart Disease:
Replace sugar with baking Splenda. Use egg substitute in place of whole eggs and eliminate the salt.
Sodium 12 mgs; **Cholesterol** 0 mgs

BLONDE BROWNIES

Ingredients:

2 cups all-purpose, unbleached flour (organic)
2 teaspoons baking powder (aluminum-free)
½ cup melted butter or low-fat margarine
2 cups packed brown sugar or Splenda brown sugar blend
2 eggs or four egg whites
1 teaspoon pure vanilla extract
1 cup chopped walnuts

Temp: 350°
Time: 20-25 minutes
Yields: 32 squares

Directions:

1. Grease a 13x9x2 baking dish, set aside.
2. Mix the melted butter and brown sugar together in a separate bowl.
3. Add the egg and vanilla.
4. Stir until well blended.
5. Sift flour with baking powder.
6. Add to first mixture and stir until all the flour is moistened.
7. Fold in chopped walnuts.
8. Place in pan.
9. Bake.
10. These brownies are chewy, they are not undercooked.

Crohn's Disease and IBS:
Finely chop or eliminate the walnuts. Use 1 cup Splenda and 1 cup brown sugar, or 2 cups Splenda brown sugar blend. Substitute 4 egg whites for the eggs.
Sugar 4 gms; **Fat** 2 gms

Diabetes:
Use 1 cup brown sugar and 1 cup Splenda, or 2 cups Splenda brown sugar blend.
Carbs 2.5 gms; **Calories** 28

Heart Disease:
Use a heart-safe margarine in place of butter. Use egg substitute in place of whole eggs. Use 1 cup brown sugar and 1 cup Splenda, or 2 cups Splenda brown sugar blend.
Sodium 9 mgs; **Cholesterol** 0 mgs

TONI'S HEALTHY LEMON SQUARES

Ingredients – Crust:
1 cup sifted cake flour (1 cup all-purpose minus 2 tablespoons)
$^1/_4$ cup confectioner's sugar
$^1/_4$ cup low-fat cream cheese
3 tablespoons canola oil

Temp: 350°
Time: 20 minutes crust;
25 minutes filling
Yields: 25 squares

Ingredients – Filling:
3 large egg whites
$^3/_4$ cup sugar or light baking Splenda
$1^1/_2$ tablespoons grated lemon zest (outside skin of lemon)
2 tablespoons all-purpose, unbleached flour (organic)
$^1/_2$ teaspoon baking powder (aluminum-free)
$^1/_4$ teaspoon salt
$^1/_3$ cup fresh lemon juice
Confectioner's sugar to dust tops (optional)

Directions – Crust:
1. Preheat oven.
2. Spray bottom of pan with cooking spray.
3. Stir together flour and confectioner's sugar.
4. With a pastry blender, cut the cream cheese into flour and sugar mixture.
5. Add the oil a little at a time and stir with a fork.
6. Press the mixture into the bottom of the baking pan.
7. Bake for about 20 minutes or until lightly brown.

Directions – Filling:
1. Beat the egg whites, lemon zest, and sugar until smooth.
2. Mix the flour, baking powder, and salt.
3. Add to the egg whites mixture and blend.
4. Mix in the lemon juice.
5. Spread over the hot crust and bake for 20 minutes.
6. Cool and cut into squares.
7. Dust with confectioner's sugar. (optional)

Crohn's Disease and IBS: Use nondairy sour cream and baking Splenda.
Sugar 6 gms; **Fat** 2 gms

Diabetes: Don't use confectioner's sugar. Use baking Splenda.
Carbs 6 gms; **Calories** 53

Heart Disease: Eliminate the salt. Replace sugar with baking Splenda.
Sodium 15 mgs; **Cholesterol** 0 mgs

HEALTHY OATMEAL CARROT BARS

Ingredients:
1/2 cup brown sugar or Splenda brown sugar blend
1/3 cup nonfat plain yogurt or unsweetened applesauce
3 egg whites
1 teaspoon pure vanilla extract
3/4 cup grated carrots
1 cup whole wheat flour (organic)
1 tablespoon baking powder (aluminum-free)
1/2 cup oatmeal
1/4 cup wheat germ
1 teaspoon cinnamon
1/2 cup raisins (optional)

Temp: 350°
Time: 30 minutes
Yields: 24 bars

Directions:
1. In a small bowl cream together applesauce, sugar, egg whites, and vanilla until light and fluffy.
2. Add the carrots and mix.
3. In a second bowl, thoroughly stir together flour, baking powder, oatmeal, wheat germ, and cinnamon.
4. Now stir the dry ingredients into the creamed mixture.
5. Fold in the raisins.
6. Pour the mixture into a canola sprayed 9x9x2 pan.
7. Bake.
8. Cool and cut into bars.

Crohn's Disease and IBS:
Replace grated carrots with baby food carrots. Omit the raisins. Use Splenda brown sugar blend.
Sugar 2 gms; **Fat** 0 gms

Diabetes:
Use Splenda brown sugar blend.
Carbs 2 gms; **Calories** 59

Heart Disease:
Use Splenda brown sugar blend.
Sodium 10 mgs; **Cholesterol** 0 mgs

BEST OATMEAL RAISIN COOKIES

Ingredients:
1 cup low-fat stick margarine*
1 cup packed brown sugar or Splenda brown sugar blend
$\frac{1}{2}$ cup granulated sugar or baking Splenda
2 eggs or 4 egg whites
1 teaspoon pure vanilla extract
$1\frac{1}{2}$ cups all-purpose, unbleached flour (organic)
1 teaspoon low-sodium baking soda
1 teaspoon cinnamon
3 cups oatmeal (can be ground)
1 cup raisins (optional)

Temp: 350°
Time: 12 minutes
Yields: 4 dozen

Directions:
1. Pre-heat oven.
2. Cream the margarine and sugar together.
3. Add the eggs and vanilla.
4. Mix in the flour, baking soda and cinnamon.
5. Stir in the oats, a cup at a time. Mix well.
6. Add the raisins.
7. Drop the batter by tablespoon onto an ungreased, shiny cookie sheet.
8. Bake cookies for about 12 minutes, or until golden brown.
9. Remove pan from the oven.
10. After a minute, remove the cookies and place on a cooling rack.

Don't use tub margarine when baking cookies, there is too much air and water whipped into it.

Crohn's Disease and IBS:
Eliminate the raisins. Use baking Splenda and egg whites.
Sugar 3 gms; **Fat** 1 gm

Diabetes:
Use baking Splenda and Splenda brown sugar blend.
Carbs 3 gms; **Calories** 20

Heart Disease:
Make the following changes: use baking Splenda, egg whites and a heart-safe margarine.
Sodium 10 mgs; **Cholesterol** 0 mgs

CHOCOLATE CHIP COOKIES

In 1939, Ruth Wakefield came up with the first chocolate chip cookie. Ruth ran out of nuts and broke up a chocolate candy bar and put it into her cookie dough.

Ingredients:
1 cup butter or low-fat stick margarine
$\frac{1}{2}$ cup packed brown sugar or Splenda brown sugar blend
1 teaspoon pure vanilla extract
2 eggs or 4 egg whites
1 teaspoon low-sodium baking soda
2$\frac{1}{4}$ cups all-purpose, unbleached flour (organic)
1$\frac{3}{4}$ cups chocolate chip morsels

Temp: 375°
Time: 10 minutes
Yields: 5 dozen

Directions:
1. Preheat oven for 10 minutes.
2. Cream together butter and sugar.
3. Add the vanilla and eggs, beat until well creamed.
4. Add the baking soda and the flour, a cup at a time. Mix well.
5. When all the dry ingredients are well mixed, add the chocolate chips.
6. Drop by tablespoons onto an ungreased, shiny cookie sheet.
7. Bake until golden brown…about 10 minutes.
8. Cool on the cookie sheet for a minute or so then place on a cooling rack.

Crohn's Disease and IBS:
Use only $\frac{1}{2}$ cup of chocolate chips and low-fat margarine. Replace 4 egg whites for the whole eggs. Use Splenda brown sugar blend.
Sugar 2 gms; **Fat** 20 gms

Diabetes:
Use Splenda brown sugar blend.
Carbs 20 gms; **Calories** 41

Heart Disease:
Use 4 egg whites in place of the 2 whole eggs. Use only $\frac{3}{4}$ cup chocolate chips. Use Splenda brown sugar blend.
Sodium 10 mgs; **Cholesterol** 0 mgs

MERINGUE KISSES

Ingredients:
3 egg whites*
¼ teaspoon cream of tartar
Pinch of salt
½ cup sugar or baking Splenda
½ teaspoon pure vanilla extract
1 (10-ounce) package semi-sweet chocolate morsels

Temp: 250°
Time: 40-45 minutes
Yields: 3 dozen

Directions:
1. Preheat oven for 10 minutes.
2. Cover cookie sheet with aluminum foil.
3. Beat egg whites with the cream of tartar and salt until it starts to get foamy.
4. Add in the sugar a little at a time until it forms peaks...about 4 minutes.
5. Fold in vanilla and chocolate morsels.
6. Place mixture by spoonfuls onto foil, about an inch apart.
7. Bake.
8. Cool completely.

Egg whites should be at room temperature before whipping.

Crohn's Disease and IBS:
Use baking Splenda and 5 ounces of chocolate morsels.
Sugar 10 gms; **Fat** 1 gm

Diabetes:
Use baking Splenda and 5 ounces chocolate morsels.
Carbs 20 gms; **Calories** 40

Heart Disease:
Eliminate the salt and use baking Splenda and 5 ounces chocolate morsels.
Sodium 0 mgs; **Cholesterol** 0 mgs

SUGAR COOKIES

Ingredients:
1 cup sugar or baking Splenda
¾ cup butter or margarine, softened
2 eggs or 4 egg whites
1 teaspoon pure vanilla extract
2½ cups all-purpose, unbleached flour (organic)
2 teaspoons baking powder (aluminum-free)*
½ teaspoon salt

Temp: 400°
Time: 6-8 Minutes
Yields: 3 Dozen

Directions:
1. Cream together sugar, shortening, eggs and vanilla.
2. Stir in remaining ingredients.
3. Cover and refrigerate at least one hour.
4. Roll dough ⅛ inch thick on a lightly floured cutting board.
5. Cut into desired shapes.
6. Place on ungreased cookie sheet.
7. Bake until lightly brown.

I use Rumford baking powder because it's aluminum-free.

Crohn's Disease and IBS:
I have Crohn's and find that too much sugar makes me ill. I use baking Splenda. If sugar is only in the recipe for sweetening, not volume, texture, or tenderness, use plain Splenda. Use 4 egg whites in place of 2 whole eggs.
Sugar 20 gms; **Fat** 1 gm

Diabetes:
Use baking Splenda.
Carbs 0 gms; **Calories** 25

Heart Disease:
Use 4 egg whites in place of the 2 whole eggs and baking Splenda. Eliminate salt.
Sodium 1 mg; **Cholesterol** 0 mgs

HAND COOKIES

This is a good rainy day project for some bonding time with your kids.

Ingredients:
Sugar cookie recipe from page 259

Temp: 400°
Time: 6-8 minutes
Yields: 15 cookies

Directions:
1. Roll dough ³/₁₆ inch thick.
2. Trace around your child's hand, (onto a piece of heavy paper), and cut out the pattern. Place pattern on dough and cut around it with a plastic knife.
3. Bake until no indentation remains when touched. (6-8 minutes)
4. Cool; decorate as desired.

Crohn's Disease and IBS:
Use baking Splenda if sugar is only in the recipe for sweetening, not volume, texture, or tenderness. Use 4 egg whites in place of 2 whole eggs.
Sugar 20 gms; **Fat** 1 gm

Diabetes:
Use baking Splenda.
Carbs 0 gms; **Calories** 25

Heart Disease:
Use 4 egg whites in place of the 2 whole eggs and baking Splenda.
Sodium 1 mg; **Cholesterol** 0 mgs

MAGIC WINDOW COOKIES

Ingredients:
Sugar cookie recipe from page 259

Temp: 375°
Time: 6-8 Minutes
Yields: 15 cookies

Directions:
1. Roll dough about ⅛ inch thick.
2. Cut out desired shapes.
3. Cut a hole in the center of the cookie with a bottle cap.
4. Make a hole in the top of the cookie with a straw.
5. Place the cut out cookie on a cookie sheet covered with aluminum foil.
6. Place a colored lifesaver into the hole in the center of the cookie.
7. Bake until the candy has melted.
8. Don't take the cookies off the cookie sheet until the cookies are completely cooled. (You can slip the foil off the cookie sheet, cookies will cool quicker.)
9. Put a string into the hole you made with the straw, and hang on the Christmas tree.

Crohn's Disease and IBS:
Use baking Splenda if sugar is only in the recipe for sweetening, not volume, texture, or tenderness. Use 4 egg whites in place of 2 whole eggs.
Sugar 20 gms; **Fat** 1 gm

Diabetes:
Use baking Splenda.
Carbs 0 gms; **Calories** 25

Heart Disease:
Use 4 egg whites in place of the 2 whole eggs and baking Splenda.
Sodium 1 mg; **Cholesterol** 0 mgs

ON THE GO BREAKFAST COOKIES

We all have those mornings when the kids get up too late and don't have time for breakfast. I have seen many children walking to school with a soda and candy bar in their hands. Give them a couple of these cookies and be assured of a nutritious breakfast substitute!

Ingredients:
½ cup butter or low-fat margarine
⅓ cup honey
1 egg or 2 egg whites
⅓ cup whole bran cereal
½ teaspoon pure orange extract
½ teaspoon orange zest
1½ teaspoons pure vanilla extract
1 cup all-purpose, unbleached flour (organic)
1 teaspoon baking powder (aluminum-free)
½ teaspoon baking soda
⅓ cup nonfat dry milk
1 cup rolled oats
½ cup raisins

Temp: 350°
Time: 10 minutes
Yields: 3 dozen

Directions:
1. Preheat oven.
2. Cream together the margarine and honey.
3. Beat in the egg.
4. Stir in the bran, rolled oats, orange juice, and vanilla.
5. Sift together the flour, baking powder, baking soda, nonfat dry milk and rolled oats.
6. Add sifted ingredients to the creamed mixture...stir well.
7. Next, stir in the raisins.
8. Grease a cookie sheet with vegetable oil spray.
9. Drop by tablespoon a full 2 inches apart on the cookie sheet.
10. Bake.

Crohn's Disease and IBS: Not recommended.
Sugar 30 gms; **Fat** 10 gms

Diabetes: Replace eggs with egg whites.
Carbs 40 gms; **Calories** 40

Heart Disease: Use 2 egg whites in place of the whole egg.
Sodium 20 mgs; **Cholesterol** 0 mgs

ANDY'S DELICIOUS QUICK AND EASY MOLASSES COOKIES

I bet you can't eat just one!

Ingredients:
3/4 cup butter or trans fat-free margarine
1 cup baking Splenda
1/4 cup molasses
1 egg or 2 egg whites
2 1/2 cups all-purpose, unbleached flour (organic)
2 teaspoons baking soda
1/2 teaspoon ginger
1 teaspoon cinnamon
pinch salt

Temp: 375°
Time: 8-10 minutes
Yields: 3 dozen

Directions:
1. Melt butter or margarine. Cool and place in mixing bowl.
2. Add sugar, molasses and eggs to butter, and mix.
3. Mix flour, baking soda and spices together and add to the mixture.
4. Chill dough. Consistency of the dough should be stiff (add a little flour if needed).
5. Roll into 1-inch balls and place 2 inches apart on a greased cookie sheet.
6. Bake.

Crohn's Disease and IBS:
Select the trans fat-free margarine. Replace egg with 2 egg whites.
Sugar 2 gms; **Fat** 3 gms

Diabetes:
Select the trans fat-free margarine. Replace egg with 2 egg whites.
Carbs 2 gms; **Calories** 7

Heart Disease:
Select a heart-safe margarine (Promise). Replace egg with 2 egg whites. Eliminate the salt.
Sodium 38 mgs; **Cholesterol** 0 mgs

SPRITZ COOKIES

This is a quick cookie for cookie swaps for holidays.

Ingredients:
1 cup butter or low-fat margarine
½ cup sugar or baking Splenda
1 egg or 2 egg whites
1 teaspoon almond or vanilla extract
½ teaspoon salt
2¼ cups unsifted, all-purpose, unbleached organic flour (Do not use self rising flour.)

Temp: 400°
Time: 6-9 minutes
Yields: 5 dozen

Directions:
1. Cream butter and sugar together.
2. Add egg and vanilla.
3. Blend in remaining ingredients.
4. Fill cookie press, form desired shapes on ungreased cookie sheet.
5. Bake 6-9 minutes or until set, but not brown.
6. To make chocolate spritz cookies, blend 2 ounces melted, unsweetened dark chocolate (cooled) into butter sugar mixture.

Crohn's Disease and IBS:
Fine to eat in moderation. Use low-fat margarine and baking Splenda. Replace egg with 2 egg whites.
Sugar 2 gms; **Fat** 1 gm

Diabetes:
Use baking Splenda.
Carbs 2 gms; **Calories** 14

Heart Disease:
Eliminate the salt and use 2 egg whites in place of the whole egg. Use a heart-safe margarine.
Sodium 0 mgs; **Cholesterol** 0 mgs

PEANUT BUTTER COOKIES

Ingredients:
½ cup butter or low-fat margarine
½ cup low-salt, low-fat peanut butter
1¼ cups all-purpose, unbleached flour (organic)
¾ cup packed brown sugar or Splenda brown sugar blend
¼ cup granulated sugar or Splenda
1 egg or 2 egg whites
1 teaspoon pure vanilla extract
½ teaspoon baking soda
½ teaspoon baking powder (aluminum-free)

Temp: 375°
Time: 8-9 minutes
Yields: 3 dozen

Directions:
1. Beat margarine and peanut butter for ½ minute using an electric mixer or food processor on medium speed.
2. Add brown sugar, granulated sugar, egg whites, vanilla, baking powder, and baking soda. Mix thoroughly.
3. Next, add ½ cup flour at a time to the mixture, until well blended.
4. Cover the dough and refrigerate until the dough is easy to handle.
5. Place 1-inch balls 2 inches apart on an ungreased shiny cookie sheet.
6. Using a fork, flatten with a crisscross motion.
7. Bake.

Crohn's Disease and IBS:
Replace eggs with 2 egg whites, Splenda in place of granulated sugar, and Splenda brown sugar blend. Use low-fat margarine.
Sugar 2 gms; **Fat** 2 gms

Diabetes:
Use Splenda in place of granulated sugar, and Splenda brown sugar blend.
Carbs 10 gms; **Calories** 10

Heart Disease:
Replace low-fat and low-salt margarine for the butter. Use the 2 egg whites, Splenda in place of granulated sugar, and Splenda brown sugar blend.
Sodium 1 mg; **Cholesterol** 0 mg

REFRIGERATOR CRISP

Ingredients:
1 cup shortening or low-fat margarine
½ cup granulated sugar or Splenda
½ cup brown sugar (packed), or Splenda brown sugar blend
1 egg or 2 egg whites
2 tablespoons reduced-fat milk
2½ cups sifted all-purpose, unbleached flour (organic)
½ teaspoon low-sodium baking soda
½ teaspoon salt
1 teaspoon cinnamon
¼ teaspoon nutmeg
¼ teaspoon cloves
½ cup finely chopped walnuts

Temp: 375°
Time: 5-7 minutes
Yields: 6 dozen

Directions:
1. Cream together shortening and sugars.
2. Add eggs and milk; beat well.
3. Sift, and then measure flour and all other dry ingredients together.
4. Stir into creamed ingredients.
5. Add chopped nuts.
6. Shape into rolls about 2½ inches in diameter.
7. Wrap in waxed paper; chill thoroughly.
8. Slice about ¼ inch thick.
9. Place 1 inch apart on lightly greased cookie sheet.
10. Bake.

Crohn's Disease and IBS:
Replace milk with nondairy milk. Use egg whites, Splenda, and Splenda brown sugar blend.
Sugar 10 gms; **Fat** 10 gms

Diabetes:
Change sugars to Splenda and Splenda brown sugar blend. Use Smart Balance for butter and margarine. Substitute milk for skim milk.
Carbs 23 gms; **Calories** 80

Heart Disease:
Replace whole egg with 2 egg whites. Eliminate salt. Use a heart-safe, low-sodium margarine.
Sodium 0 mgs; **Cholesterol** 0 mgs

PEANUT BUTTER RICE KRISPIE SQUARES

Ingredients:

6 cups Rice Krispies

2 tablespoons canola oil or trans fat-free margarine

1 (10-ounce) package marshmallows (40 regular or 4 cups miniature)

2 tablespoons low-fat peanut butter

Temp: Low
Time: 2 minutes
Yields: 24 squares

Directions:

1. Place canola oil, or margarine, in a large saucepan over low heat.
2. Add marshmallows and peanut butter. Stir using a wooden spoon until completely melted.
3. Remove pan from heat.
4. Add Rice Krispies and stir until coated with the marshmallow peanut butter mixture.
5. Using a buttered spatula, press evenly into a 13x9x2 pan coated with cooking spray.

Crohn's Disease and IBS:
Enjoy!
Sugar 20 gms; **Fat** 3 gms

Diabetes:
Enjoy!
Carbs 30 gms; **Calories** 150

Heart Disease:
Enjoy!
Sodium 200 mgs; **Cholesterol** 0 mgs

PIES

The most important factor to remember in making tender flaky pie crust is to work quickly and not handle the dough too much. One summer while in college, I worked on a lobster bake. One of my jobs was to make 12 blueberry and 12 apple pies every day. The pies came out great, because I didn't have time to fuss with the crust.

The secret to making perfect pie crust is described in the following recipe for a standard Pastry two-crust pie.

INGREDIENTS: (For a 9" pie)
2 cups all-purpose, unbleached flour (organic)
1 teaspoon salt
$^2/_3$ cup plus 2 tablespoons shortening
cold water (approximately $^1/_4$ cup)

DIRECTIONS:
1. Sift and measure flour.
2. Mix in salt.
3. Cut in shortening with a pastry blender or two knives used in a scissors fashion until lumps are the size of giant peas. The pastry should have streaks of shortening running through it.
4. Sprinkle with water until all the mixture is moist. Gently toss the mixture with a fork.
5. Gather dough and press into a ball. Divide dough in half for two-crust pie.
6. Next, lightly flour rolling pin and board.
7. Roll dough by gently working from the center to the outer edge in all directions, lifting the rolling pin as you get to the edge. This will prevent thin edges that split and break.
8. Don't turn pastry over when rolling it out, gently move pastry around brushing a little flour under pastry if it seems to stick. Too much flour makes tough pie crust.
9. Roll pastry about $^1/_8$" thick.
10. When the pastry is a round circle 1" larger (all around) than the inverted pie plate, place pastry in the pie plate.
11. Don't stretch the pastry over the edge of the plate, it will shrink when it is baked.
12. Prepare filling and place into the pastry-lined pan.
13. Prepare top crust the same as the bottom one.
14. Fold pastry in half, make steam vents.
15. Place pastry evenly over filling.
16. Moisten the edge of the lower edge to help seal pastry together.
17. Fold edge of top pastry under the bottom one and make appropriate edges.
18. Brush top of pie with one of the following toppings.

TOPPINGS

    A. Whole whipped egg for a glazed top

    B. Milk makes a shiny top

    C. Water or milk and sprinkle of sugar yield a sugary top. (Good for tart pies)

STEAM VENTS

For berry pies, make an O Hole in the center with large macaroni inserted to prevent bubbling over.

EDGES

A) Used for one or two-crust pies

1. **Fork** – Using a fork, press gently around the edge of the pie crust.

2. **Fluted** – Make stand-up edge. With right index finger on the inside and the left index and thumb on the outside, pinch.

B) Used for one-crust pies

1. **Penny** – Cut circles the size of a penny. I use a vanilla bottle cap. Trim bottom pastry even with pie plate. Brush edge with water, and place circles overlapping each other all around the rim. Seal each with water.

2. **Braid** – make three equal strips of pastry dough and braid. Seal onto crust with water.

HINTS

1. In making a one-crust pie shell, be sure to prick the bottom of the pie shell sufficiently, before baking. It will keep the crust from bubbling up.

2. For best results, whip egg whites at room temperature; you will get more volume.

3. Too much sugar will cause meringues to get beady.

4. Make small tarts with extra pastry.

5. Make up a number of pies and freeze them. (It saves money.)

6. Make a pie out of leftover stew; it's a pleasant change.

RHUBARB PIE

Ingredients:
Pastry for a 2-crust pie (page 268)
4 cups unpeeled rhubarb (cut into 1-inch pieces)
1½ cups Splenda or sugar
6 tablespoons all-purpose, unbleached flour (organic)
Dash of salt
1⅓ tablespoons butter or trans fat-free margarine.

Temp: 450°
Time: 15 minutes then,
        350° for 45 minutes
Yields: 8 pieces

Directions:
1. Mix 2 tablespoons of the flour with 2 tablespoons of the sugar and sprinkle over bottom of pastry in a 9″ pie plate. Add rhubarb to pie plate.
2. Mix the remaining flour and sugar together, sprinkle over the rhubarb.
3. Add dash of salt.
4. Dot with margarine.
5. Place top crust over filling and flute edges.
6. Follow pastry procedure on page 268.
7. Bake.

Crohn's Disease and IBS:
Not recommended.
Sugar 2 gms; **Fat** 8 gms

Diabetes:
Use Splenda in place of the sugar. Substitute Smart Balance for margarine.
Carbs 7 gms; **Calories** 88

Heart Disease:
Replace butter with a heart-safe margarine, sugar with Splenda. Eliminate the salt.
Sodium 16 mgs; **Cholesterol** 0 mgs

PUMPKIN OR SQUASH PIE

Ingredients:

1 (9-inch) unbaked pie shell, or make your own (page 268)
15 ounces canned or cooked pumpkin or squash
$\frac{1}{2}$ cup sugar or Splenda
$\frac{1}{2}$ teaspoon salt
$\frac{1}{2}$ teaspoon cinnamon
1 teaspoon ginger
$\frac{1}{4}$ teaspoon nutmeg
3 tablespoons molasses
2 eggs slightly beaten or egg substitute
1 cup low-fat milk

Temp: 425° *– 15 min.*
350° – 25 min.
Time: 40-45 minutes
Yields: 6 servings

Directions:

1. Mix pumpkin or squash, sugar, salt, cinnamon, ginger, nutmeg and molasses.
2. Add beaten eggs and milk. Mix thoroughly.
3. Pour into unbaked pie shell.
4. Bake.

Crohn's Disease and IBS:
Use a nondairy milk. Replace sugar with Splenda and eggs with 4 egg whites.
Sugar 6 gms; **Fat** 3 gms

Diabetes:
Change the granulated sugar to Splenda. Use skim milk.
Carbs 3 gms; **Calories** 43

Heart Disease:
Eliminate the salt. Either use egg substitute or 4 egg whites (two egg whites equal one whole egg).
Sodium 9 mgs; **Cholesterol** 0 mgs

BEST APPLE PIE

I found this recipe in a country wallpaper book, and it is the best apple pie.

Ingredients:
Pastry for a 2-crust pie (page 268)
6 or 7 cups pared sliced apples
$1/4$ cup granulated sugar or Splenda
$1/4$ teaspoon salt
$3/4$ to 1 teaspoon cinnamon
$1/4$ cup light brown sugar or Splenda brown sugar blend
1 tablespoon butter or trans fat-free margarine

Temp: 425°
Time: 40 minutes: lower temperature to 325° and cook more if needed (about 20 minutes)
Yields: 6 servings

Directions:
1. Pre-heat oven.
2. Prepare pastry for a two-crust pie.
3. Wash, peel, and core apples. Slice thin.
4. Combine sugar, salt, and cinnamon.
5. Sprinkle mixture over sliced apples.
6. Place apples in pastry-lined pie shell.
7. Dot top of the apples with butter.
8. Place top pastry over filling.
9. Make steam vents and flute edge. Glaze top of crust with whole whipped egg.
10. Bake.

I use Macintosh apples so I'll need less sugar. They are naturally sweet.

Crohn's Disease and IBS:
Replace sugars with Splenda and Splenda brown sugar blend, and butter with a trans fat-free margarine.
Sugar 10 gms; **Fat** 2 gms

Diabetes:
Use Splenda in place of granulated sugar. Use a trans fat-free margarine.
Carbs 19 carbs; **Calories** 83

Heart Disease:
Eliminate salt. Use a heart-safe margarine. Replace sugar with Splenda.
Sodium 11 mgs; **Cholesterol** 0 mgs

YUMMY STRAWBERRY PEACH PIE

Ingredients:
3 cups thinly sliced fresh peaches
1 cup sliced fresh sweet strawberries
²/₃ cup sugar or Splenda
Pinch salt
2 tablespoons all-purpose, unbleached flour (organic)
1 tablespoon margarine or butter
Few drops lemon juice
Pastry for a 2-crust pie (see page 268)

Temp: 425°
Time: 40 minutes
Yields: 6 servings

Directions:
1. Place the lower crust into a 9-inch pie plate.
2. Blend sugar, salt, and flour in a small mixing bowl.
3. Mix lightly with sliced peaches and strawberries.
4. Fill bottom crust with the fruit filling.
5. Dot top of filling with margarine or butter.
6. Place top crust over filling and flute the edges.
7. Beat one egg and brush on top crust to give it a golden color.
8. Cut steam vent on top crust.
9. Bake.
10. Cool and serve.

Crohn's Disease and IBS:
Use trans fat-free margarine and Splenda.
Sugar 8 gms; **Fat** 2 gms

Diabetes:
Use trans fat-free margarine and Splenda.
Carbs 10 carbs; **Calories** 38

Heart Disease:
Eliminate the salt. Use Promise margarine and Splenda.
Sodium 0 mgs; **Cholesterol** 0 mgs

SWEET POTATO PIE

Recipe from a Southern friend.

Ingredients:
2 egg yolks
1¹/₂ cups mashed sweet potato
¹/₂ cup brown sugar or Splenda brown sugar blend
¹/₂ teaspoon salt
1 teaspoon cinnamon
¹/₂ teaspoon nutmeg
³/₄ cup low-fat milk
2 beaten egg whites

Temp: 400° F
Time: 45 minutes
Yields: 6 servings

Directions:
1. Combine egg yolks, sweet potato, brown sugar, salt, and spices.
2. Blend in milk and beaten egg whites.
3. Pour into a 9-inch pastry-lined pie plate.
4. Bake.

Crohn's Disease and IBS:
Use nondairy milk. Replace egg yolks with egg substitute. Use Splenda brown sugar blend and Splenda.
Sugar 4 gms; **Fat** 1 gm

Diabetes:
Use Splenda brown sugar blend. Use egg substitute in place of egg yolks.
Carbs 12 gms; **Calories** 34

Heart Disease:
Eliminate the salt. Replace egg yolks with egg substitute.
Sodium 18 mgs; **Carbohydrates** 3 mgs

MRS. WYMAN'S LEMON SPONGE PIE

Ingredients:
¼ cup soft butter or low-fat, low-salt margarine
1 cup sugar or Splenda
3 eggs separated
3 tablespoons all-purpose, unbleached flour (organic)
6 tablespoons lemon juice, and 1 teaspoon grated lemon rind
2 cups low-fat milk
Pinch cream of tartar
Enough pastry for a 10-inch pie plate (See one-crust oil pastry recipe on next page.)

Temp: 425° for 15 minutes,
then 325° for 25 minutes
Yields: 6 servings

Directions:
1. Beat separated egg whites until they form a peak, set aside.
2. Mix together ¼ cup of the sugar and the cream of tartar.
3. Cream margarine and remaining sugar, add to sugar mixture.
4. Add egg yolks to the mixture and beat.
5. Next add flour, lemon juice, and rind.
6. Pour in milk.
7. Lastly fold in the beaten egg whites.
8. Place mixture into the unbaked pastry shell.
9. Bake.

Crohn's Disease and IBS:
Use nondairy milk and egg substitute. Also use the Splenda in place of sugar.
Sugar 25 gms; **Fat** 6 gms

Diabetes:
Use Splenda.
Carbs 4 gms; **Calories** 49

Heart Disease:
Use AHA recommended margarine. Use egg substitute in place of the egg yolks. Beat the egg whites and fold into the mixture.
Sodium 30 mgs; **Cholesterol** 1 mg

ONE-CRUST OIL PASTRY

This crust is a healthier alternative to crust made with solid shortening.
My friend Julie Mullen uses this crust with her Blueberry Glacé Pie.
(See recipe for Blueberry Glacé Pie on page 277.)

Ingredients:
2 cups all-purpose, unbleached flour (organic)
2-3 pinches baking powder (aluminum-free)
2/3 cup vegetable oil (canola)
Pinch salt
1/3 cup orange juice

Temp: 450°
Time: 12-15 minutes
Yields: 1 pie shell

Directions:
1. Mix flour, oil, and salt until particles are the size of small peas.
2. Add orange juice a tablespoon at a time until the pastry forms a ball.
3. If pastry seems dry add a little more oil, not water.
4. Roll the pastry at least 2 inches larger than the pie plate.
5. Use the coin edging as described on page 269.
6. Bake.

Crohn's Disease and IBS:
Use egg substitute in place of eggs. Use a nondairy milk.
Sugar 1 gm; **Fat** 5 gms

Diabetes:
Substitute flour with rice flour.
Carbs 4 gms; **Calories** 70

Heart Disease:
Eliminate the salt and use egg substitute.
Sodium 27 mgs; **Cholesterol** 0 mgs

MULLEN'S BLUEBERRY GLACÉ PIE

My friends the Mullens are teachers in Maine and also grow many acres of wild blueberries each summer. Wild Maine blueberries are small and sweet.

Ingredients:
3 cups blueberries
³/₄ cup of water
1 tablespoon butter or trans fat-free margarine
1 cup sugar or baking Splenda
3 tablespoons cornstarch
Pinch of salt

Temp: Medium heat, stove top
Time: 10 minutes
Yields: 6 servings

Directions:
1. In ³/₄ cup of water, gently boil 1 cup blueberries and 1 tablespoon butter for 4 minutes.
2. In a separate bowl, mix 1 cup sugar, 3 tablespoons cornstarch, and a dash of salt.
3. Add dry mixture to hot blueberry mixture, stirring constantly.
4. Cook slowly until thick and clear, then remove from heat.
5. Pour 2 cups raw blueberries into mixture and mix gently.
6. Turn into 9-inch baked pie shell and refrigerate. (see recipe on page 276)

Delicious and full of antioxidants!!!!!!

Crohn's Disease and IBS:
Blend blueberries in the food processor. Use Splenda in place of sugar. Use a trans fat-free margarine.
Sugar 5 gms; **Fat** 2 gms

Diabetes:
Replace sugar with Splenda, it's only used to sweeten. Use a trans fat-free margarine.
Carbs 10 gms; **Calories** 40

Heart Disease:
Replace sugar with Splenda. Eliminate salt. Use a heart-safe margarine (Promise).
Sodium 10 mgs; **Cholesterol** 0 mgs

NEW YORK STYLE CHEESECAKE

Ingredients:
Graham cracker crumbs
   (Enough to coat the buttered spring form pan)
1 pound small curd low-fat cottage cheese
2 (8-ounce) packages low-fat cream cheese
1½ cups granulated sugar or Splenda
4 eggs, slightly beaten or egg substitute
⅓ cup cornstarch
2 tablespoons lemon juice
1 teaspoon pure vanilla extract
½ cup melted Smart Balance margarine
1 pint low-fat sour cream or yogurt

Temp: 325°
Time: 1 hour 10 minutes,
          2 hours in with no heat
Yields: 12 servings

Directions:
1. Grease 1 (9-inch) spring form pan; coat with the graham cracker crumbs.
2. Mix all the above ingredients in a food processor until well blended.
3. If you don't have a food processor, mix with an electric blender one ingredient at a time until well blended.
4. Pour into prepared pan.
5. Bake for 1 hour, 10 minutes in a 325° F oven until firm.
6. Turn off oven and let the cheesecake stand in the oven for 2 hours.
7. Remove from oven and cool completely on a wire rack.
8. Chill.
9. Remove the sides of the spring form pan.

This cheesecake may be frozen.

Crohn's Disease and IBS:
Not recommended.
Sugar 10 gms; **Fat** 3 gms

Diabetes:
Replace eggs with egg substitute. Use Splenda, it's only used as a sweetener. Check with your doctor before eating.
Carbs 2 gms; **Calories** 66

Heart Disease:
Check with your doctor before eating. Replace eggs with an egg substitute. Use Splenda and a heart-safe margarine.
Sodium 90 mgs; **Cholesterol** 0 mgs

GEMAINE'S PUMPKIN PUDDING

Ingredients:
$^1/_4$ cup soft butter or trans fat-free margarine
$^1/_2$ teaspoon cinnamon
Pinch of salt
1 cup pumpkin, mashed
$^1/_2$ cup sugar or baking Splenda
$^1/_2$ teaspoon nutmeg
3 eggs, beaten or egg substitute

Temp: 375°
Time: 40 minutes
Yields: 6 servings

Directions:
1. Cream margarine and sugar.
2. Blend in spices and salt.
3. Add beaten eggs and pumpkin.
4. Bake. Serve cold or hot with whipped cream. (In a greased 1$^1/_2$ quart baking dish).

Crohn's Disease and IBS:
Replace eggs with egg substitute. Use baking Splenda in place of sugar. Use a nondairy milk substitute.
Sugar 17 gms; **Fat** 6 gms

Diabetes:
Use baking Splenda in place of sugar. Instead of butter, use a trans fat-free margarine.
Carbs 18 gms; **Calories** 70

Heart Disease:
Replace eggs with egg substitute and margarine with a heart-safe margarine. Eliminate the salt. Use Splenda in place of sugar.
Sodium 47 mgs; **Cholesterol** 0 mgs

JULIE'S BREAD PUDDING

This was the recipe my students and I made for the soup kitchen.

Ingredients:
6 slices whole wheat bread (toasted)
¼ cup sugar or Splenda
¼ cup brown sugar or Splenda brown sugar blend
1 teaspoon cinnamon
⅓ cup raisins (optional)
2 eggs or egg substitute
1 teaspoon pure vanilla extract
2 cups low-fat milk scalded
¼ cup butter or trans fat-free margarine

Temp: 350°
Time: 45 minutes
Yields: 6-8 servings

Directions:
1. Preheat oven.
2. Toast bread.
3. Cut toast into cubes and place into a 1½-inch deep greased casserole dish.
4. In a bowl, mix the eggs, sugar, cinnamon, and vanilla.
5. Next, slowly add the scalded milk and melted margarine to the egg mixture.
6. Pour the mixture over the bread and add the raisins.
7. Place casserole dish in a square 9x9x2 pan. Pour 1 inch of hot water into the pan.
8. Bake until a knife inserted comes out clean.

Crohn's Disease and IBS:
Use a nondairy milk. I use soy. Eliminate raisins. Use Splenda. Change whole eggs to egg substitute.
Sugar 10 gms; **Fat** 3 gms

Diabetes:
Use gluten-free bread. Replace sugars with Splenda.
Carbs 6 gms; **Calories** 10

Heart Disease:
Replace the eggs with egg substitute. Use Splenda and a heart-safe margarine. Use a sodium-free bread. Change whole eggs to egg substitute.
Sodium 31 mgs; **Cholesterol** 1 mg

TAPIOCA PUDDING

Ingredients:
1 egg white
3 tablespoons sugar or Splenda
1 egg yolk
2 cups low-fat milk
3 tablespoons quick cooking tapioca
2 tablespoons sugar or Splenda (to use with the egg white)
Pinch of salt
$\frac{1}{2}$ teaspoon pure vanilla extract

Temp: Medium
Time: Cook until thick
Yields: 4 servings

Directions:
1. Separate the egg. Place whites in a separate bowl, ready for beating.
2. Add 2 tablespoons of the 2 cups of milk to the egg yolk and beat.
3. Place the remaining milk in saucepan. Add sugar, tapioca, and salt.
4. Heat mixture slowly, to the boiling point.
5. Add beaten egg yolk and milk. Cook until it thickens, stirring frequently.
6. Beat the egg white until stiff.
7. Add the 2 tablespoons sugar and continue beating until the whites hold up in peaks.
8. Pour the hot thickened tapioca over the beaten egg white. The hotter this mixture and the faster you add it, the better.
9. Beat mixture until smooth.
10. Add vanilla and pour into serving dishes.

Crohn's Disease and IBS:
Use nondairy milk and Splenda. Replace whole eggs with 2 egg whites.
Sugar 3 gms; **Fat** 1 gm

Diabetes:
Use Splenda for sugar. Use skim milk.
Carbs 12 gms; **Calories** 70

Heart Disease:
Eliminate the salt. Replace whole eggs with 2 egg whites. Use skim milk and Splenda for refined sugar.
Sodium 13 mgs; **Cholesterol** 51 mgs

GRAPENUT PUDDING

Ingredients:
2 cups scalded low-fat milk
½ cup Grape Nuts
6 tablespoons sugar or Splenda
2 well beaten eggs or egg substitute
Pinch salt
1 teaspoon pure vanilla extract (taste better)
Dot with butter or trans fat-free margarine

Temp: 375°
Time: 30 minutes
Yields: 4 servings

Directions:
1. Scald milk. Add grape nuts and allow to soak for 10 minutes.
2. Beat eggs; add sugar, vanilla and milk to mixture.
3. Dot with butter.
4. Bake.

Crohn's Disease and IBS:
Soak the Grape Nuts in warm water before using. Use a nondairy milk and Splenda. Use a trans fat-free margarine.
Sugar 7 gms; **Fat** 1 gm

Diabetes:
Replace egg with an egg substitute. Substitute Splenda for sugar. Use a trans fat-free margarine.
Carbs 18 gms; **Calories** 70

Heart Disease:
Replace butter with a heart-safe margarine. Use Splenda in place of the sugar. Use an egg substitute. Eliminate salt.
Sodium 126 mgs; **Cholesterol** 2 mgs

BROWN SUGAR PUDDING

This is one of my husband's favorite treats, handed down from his Canadian grandmother. Best served warm with a scoop of vanilla ice cream or frozen yogurt.

Ingredients – Bottom Dough:
½ cup sugar or baking Splenda
1 tablespoon light butter or trans fat-free margarine
1 cup fat-free milk
2 cups all-purpose, unbleached flour (organic)
2 teaspoons baking powder (aluminum-free)
1 teaspoon pure vanilla extract
Pinch salt

Temp: 375°
Time: 30 to 40 minutes
Yields: 6 servings

Ingredients – Top Syrup:
2 cups brown sugar or Splenda brown sugar blend
2 cups water
1 tablespoon light butter or trans fat-free margarine
1 teaspoon pure vanilla extract

Directions:
1. Cream the sugar, butter and vanilla in a medium size mixing bowl.
2. Add salt and baking powder to the mixture.
3. Alternately add milk and flour.
4. Pour batter into a greased, square 8x8x2 cake pan.
5. Combine the brown sugar, water, and margarine in a saucepan and boil for 3-5 minutes.
6. Add 1 teaspoon vanilla to mixture.
7. Pour mixture over the batter.
8. Bake.

Crohn's Disease and IBS:
Replace milk with nondairy milk. Use Splenda brown sugar blend. Replace butter with a trans fat-free margarine.
Sugar 2 gms; **Fat** 4 gms

Diabetes:
Replace milk with nondairy milk. Use Splenda brown sugar blend. Replace butter with a trans fat-free margarine.
Carbs 1 gm; **Calories** 42

Heart Disease:
Replace milk with nondairy milk. Eliminate salt. Use Splenda brown sugar blend. Replace butter with a heart-safe margarine.
Sodium 30 mgs; **Cholesterol** 0 mgs

DURGIN PARK INDIAN PUDDING

Durgin Park "The famed 18th century Faneuil Hall Marketplace" Boston, MA. This is a recipe I used to make for lobster bakes on Indian Island, in Maine.

Ingredients:
3 cups scalded, low-fat milk, divided
1¼ cup dark molasses
2 tablespoons sugar or Splenda
2 tablespoons butter or trans fat-free margarine
¼ teaspoon salt
⅛ teaspoon baking powder (aluminum-free)
1 egg or egg substitute
½ cup yellow cornmeal

Temp: 450° until it boils
then 300° for remaining time
Time: 5-7 hours
Yields: 6 servings

Directions:
1. Preheat oven to 450°.
2. Mix 1½ cups milk with the molasses, sugar, butter, salt, baking powder, egg and cornmeal in a medium mixing bowl.
3. Pour the mixture into a well-greased stone crock, (or casserole dish) and bake until it boils.
4. Stir in the other 1½ cups milk.
5. Next, lower the oven temperature to 300° and bake.
6. Serve warm with ice cream or frozen yogurt.

Crohn's Disease and IBS:
Use a nondairy milk and an egg substitute. Use a trans fat-free margarine and Splenda.
Sugar 9 gms; **Fat** 1 gm

Diabetes:
Replace eggs with egg substitute. Use skim milk and Splenda.
Carbs 28 gms; **Calories** 146

Heart Disease:
Eliminate salt and use a pinch of ginger in its place. Ginger aids in digestion. Replace eggs with an egg substitute. Use skim milk and Splenda.
Sodium 90 mgs; **Cholesterol** 4 mgs

RICE PUDDING

Ingredients:
2 cups water
$\frac{1}{2}$ cup uncooked rice
$\frac{1}{2}$ teaspoon salt
$\frac{1}{2}$ cup raisins
1 tablespoons butter or trans fat-free margarine
2 cups instant nonfat milk
$\frac{1}{2}$ cup sugar or baking Splenda
1 cup warm water
1 teaspoon pure vanilla extract

Temp: Boiling
Time: 30 minutes
Yields: 6 servings

Directions:
1. Boil 2 cups of water.
2. Add rice, salt, raisins, and margarine.
3. Lower heat, until just bubbling, cover and cook 30 minutes.
4. Remove from heat.
5. Mix dry milk, sugar and 1 cup water.
6. Pour the milk mixture into the rice.
7. Cook thoroughly over low heat.
8. Add vanilla.

Chocolate leaves will add a special touch to your puddings. Wash and dry either artificial or nonpoisonous leaves. (Rose leaves are good.) Melt semisweet chocolate over a double boiler. With a small brush or spatula, paint the melted chocolate to the underside of the leaves. Place the leaves on a cookie sheet with the chocolate side up. Cool leaves in the refrigerator until they get firm. To remove the leaves, gently pull them apart. Use these chocolate leaves to garnish your puddings and desserts.

Crohn's Disease and IBS:
Eliminate the raisins. Change butter to trans fat-free margarine, whole milk to nondairy milk, and refined sugar to baking Splenda.
Sugar 11 gms; **Fat** 1 gm

Diabetes:
Use Smart Balance margarine. Use baking Splenda. Replace whole milk with skim milk.
Carbs 9 gms; **Calories** 50

Heart Disease:
Eliminate salt. Use a heart-safe margarine. Change whole milk to skim milk. Replace refined sugar with baking Splenda.
Sodium 35 mgs; **Cholesterol** 1 mg

COMMON ABBREVIATIONS AND MEASUREMENTS

teaspoon = tsp = t
Tablespoon = Tbsp = T
Cup = c
Ounce = oz
Pint = pt
Quart = qt
Gallon = gal
Pound = lb
Peck = pk
Dash = pinch or less than $1/8$ tsp

3 teaspoons = 1 tablespoon
5 tablespoons + 1 teaspoon = $1/3$ cup
4 tablespoons = $1/4$ cup
16 tablespoons = 1 cup
1 cup = 8 fluid ounces
2 cups = 1 pint
4 cups = 1 quart = 32 ounces
1 pound = 16 ounces (dry measure)

Liquid Measures

1 cup = 8 fluid ounces = $1/2$ pint = 237 ml
2 cups = 16 fluid ounces = 1 pint = 474 ml
4 cups = 32 fluid ounces = 1 quart = 946 ml
2 pints = 32 fluid ounces= 1 quart = .964 liters
4 quarts = 128 fluid ounces = 1 gallon = 3.784 liters
8 quarts = one peck
4 pecks = one bushel
Dash = less than $1/4$ teaspoon

Dry Measures

3 teaspoons = 1 tablespoon = $1/2$ ounce = 14.3 grams
2 tablespoons = $1/8$ cup = 1 fluid ounce = 28.3 grams
4 tablespoons = $1/4$ cup = 2 fluid ounces = 56.7 grams
$5 1/3$ tablespoons = $1/3$ cup = 2.6 fluid ounces = 75.6 grams
8 tablespoons = $1/2$ cup = 4 ounces = 113.4 grams = 1 stick butter
12 tablespoons = $3/4$ cup = 6 ounces = .375 pound = 170 grams
32 tablespoons = 2 cups = 16 ounces = 1 pound = 453.6 grams
64 tablespoons = 4 cups = 32 ounces = 2 pounds = 907 grams

COMMON COOKING SUBSTITUTES

1 teaspoon baking powder = $1/4$ teaspoon baking soda plus $1/2$ teaspoon cream of tartar

1 square unsweetened chocolate = 3 tablespoons unsweetened cocoa powder plus 1 tablespoon vegetable oil

1 cup applesauce = 1 cup canola oil

1 tablespoon cornstarch (as a thickener) = 2 tablespoons all-purpose flour

1 cup cake flour = 1 cup all-purpose flour, minus 2 tablespoons

1 cup mayonnaise = 1 cup no-fat yogurt

$1/2$ cup brown sugar = 2 tablespoons molasses into $1/2$ cup granulated sugar

1 cup granulated sugar = 1 cup Splenda

1 cup sour or buttermilk = 1 tablespoon lemon juice plus 1% whole milk to equal 1 cup

COOKING AND FOOD TERMS

Baked	Dry heat cooking in an oven.
Baste	Spooning pan juices over food, as it is cooking.
Beat	Making a mixture smooth by whipping with a whisk or mixer.
Blanch	To partially cook vegetables in boiling water.
Blend	Combining ingredients to become one.
Boil	To heat a liquid, which causes it to produce bubbles that rise and break the surface of the liquid.
Braise	To brown meat, and then cook it slowly in a small amount of water in a covered pan. Works best for tough meat.
Broil	To cook food under a direct source of intense heat.
Chop	Using a sharp knife to cut food into smaller pieces.
Clarified Butter	Heat the butter until solids and foam appear. Skim off the foam and discard solids. Pour the yellow liquid into a clean jar (clarified butter). A clear residue will remain, discard it. Clarified butter will not burn like solid butter does.
Cream	To beat shortening or butter with sugar until smooth and well blended. Cut in using two knives or a pastry blender to work solid shortening into dry ingredients. Example: biscuits or pie crust.
Dash	A dash is about 1/16 of a teaspoon.
De-glaze	Pouring a small amount of liquid into a hot pan in which something has been cooked. To dislodge cooked on food bits from the bottom of the pan to be used for gravy.
Drain	Using a strainer to remove the unwanted liquid in a pan.
Dredge	The process of coating food with flour before cooking.
Fold	To gently combine a light, airy mixture with a heavier mixture. The heavier mixture that is placed on the bottom is lifted from the bottom with a rubber scraper and blended into the lighter mixture.
Grate	Shredding solid food against the sharp holes of a grater.
Julienne	To cut food into thin two inch strips.
Knead	To mix dough with the palms of your hands until the dough is smooth.

Leaven	Yeast, baking soda or baking powder is used to cause batters and dough to rise.
Mince	To cut into very small pieces (minced garlic).
Mix	To combine foods until they are well blended.
To Proof-Yeast	The process of testing the freshness of yeast. Add yeast to water with a tablespoon of sugar and wait to see if bubbles form. If bubbles form, the yeast is good. If no bubbles form, you start over again with new yeast.
Pre-heat	Allowing the oven to heat to the desired temperature (10 minutes).
Puree	Blending food until it becomes liquid.
Reduce	Liquid is boiled away to make a stew richer and thicker. It makes the liquid more concentrated.
Sauté	Cooking in a pan, over direct heat, with little or no fat.
Sift	Placing dry ingredients into a sifter to incorporate air, remove lumps, and thoroughly mix the ingredients. There are 2 extra tablespoons of flour in unsifted flour.
Zest	The outer skin of the citrus fruits (lemon, lime, orange).

DEFINITIONS OF TERMS USED IN THIS COOKBOOK

Aluminum-Free Baking Powder
Only contains three ingredients: baking soda, cornstarch, and calcium acid phosphate. There are some baking powders that contain a fourth ingredient, sodium aluminum sulfite. I find the aluminum leaves a bitter taste. This ingredient is added to delay the reaction between the baking powder and water. The safety of aluminum is still not proven. When using aluminum-free baking powder, mix all the dry ingredients together and then add them to the liquid ingredients. Don't over mix.

Antioxidants   Fight toxic compounds, such as free radicals in the body. Free radicals may damage unsaturated fatty acids, and DNA. It is thought that free radicals may contribute to many diseases, such as cancer, heart disease, aging, hardening of the arteries. Antioxidants are found in fruits and vegetables.

Beta-carotene   Prevents oxidation and enhances the immune system. It is believed to prevent heart disease and cancer. Have diets rich in fruits and vegetables.

Carbohydrates   They vary from simple sugars to complex starches. They provide 4 calories per gram.

Carotenoids   They give vegetables and fruits their color (red, orange and deep yellow). Broccoli and dark green vegetables are also a source of carotenoids. They provide us with beta-carotene.

Cholesterol   It's a fat-like substance only found in animal food. Too much clogs the arteries. HDL is the good cholesterol and LDL is the bad cholesterol.

Cruciferous   Vegetables, such as, broccoli, cabbage, Brussels sprouts, turnip, and rutabagas. There are cancer-fighting chemicals called indoles in these vegetables.

Dietary fats   Fats provide 9 calories per gram.

Dietary Fiber   The parts of the fruits and vegetables that can't be digested. Studies show that diets high in fiber are great in reducing certain cancers and heart disease. Your diet should be high in fiber.

Ethylene Gas   A colorless gas that stimulates ripening in fruits and vegetables.

Folic Acid   Known as a Folate, a B vitamin that is involved in protein metabolism. It works mainly in the brain and nervous system. It's found in green leafy vegetables.

Free Radicals   Toxic molecules of oxygen that damage areas of our bodies. Limit exposure and increase your ability to apprehend them with foods rich in antioxidants. Some causes of free radicals are exposure to smoke, excessive heat or cold, alcohol, sunburn, lack of clean air, stress, power line wires, TV, computers, synthetic materials, preservatives, environmental pollution. These are only a few, there are more. You can fight these free radicals by including more antioxidants in your diet. The antioxidants are listed in this book.

Fructose   A simple sugar found in fruits.

Ischemic Stroke   This stroke occurs when an artery in the brain or neck becomes blocked.

Nutraceutical   Natural bioactive chemical compounds that have health promoting properties. They are believed to prevent and cure diseases.

Organic   Agricultural foods grown naturally with no pesticides. They protect our environment. Organically grown foods may be more expensive but are the healthier choice.

Phytochemical   A natural plant substance that works with nutrients and dietary fiber to protect against disease, such as cancer, heart disease, strokes, high blood pressure, and urinary tract infections.

RECIPE INDEX

RECIPE INDEX

294